T0226964

Geriatric Syndromes

Editors

JENNIFER KIM
SALLY MILLER

NURSING CLINICS
OF NORTH AMERICA

www.nursing.theclinics.com

Consulting Editor
STEPHEN D. KRAU

September 2017 • Volume 52 • Number 3

ELSEVIER

1600 John F. Kennedy Boulevard ● Suite 1800 ● Philadelphia, Pennsylvania, 19103-2899

http://www.theclinics.com

NURSING CLINICS OF NORTH AMERICA Volume 52, Number 3
September 2017 ISSN 0029-6465, ISBN-13: 978-0-323-54560-0

Editor: Kerry Holland
Developmental Editor: Casey Potter

Nursing Clinics of North America (ISSN 0029-6465) is published quarterly by Elsevier Inc., 360 Park Avenue South, New York, NY 10010-1710. Months of issue are March, June, September, and December. Periodicals postage paid at New York, NY and additional mailing offices. Subscription price per year is, $155.00 (US individuals), $465.00 (US institutions), $275.00 (international individuals), $567.00 (international institutions), $220.00 (Canadian individuals), $567.00 (Canadian institutions), $100.00 (US students), and $135.00 (international students). To receive student/resident rate, orders must be accompanied by name of affiliated institution, date of term, and the signature of program/residency coordinator on institution letterhead. Orders will be billed at individual rate until proof of status is received. Foreign air speed delivery is included in all *Clinics* subscription prices. All prices are subject to change without notice. **POSTMASTER:** Send address changes to *Nursing Clinics*, Elsevier Health Sciences Division, Subscription Customer Service, 3251 Riverport Lane, Maryland Heights, MO 63043. **Customer Service: Telephone: 1-800-654-2452** (U.S. and Canada); **1-314-447-8871 (outside U.S. and Canada). Fax: 1-314-447-8029. E-mail: journalscustomerservice-usa@elsevier.com** (for print support) and **journalsonlinesupport-usa@elsevier.com** (for online support).

Nursing Clinics of North America is covered in *EMBASE/Excerpta Medica, MEDLINE/PubMed (Index Medicus), Social Sciences Citation Index, Current Contents, ASCA, Cumulative Index to Nursing, RNdex Top 100,* and Allied Health Literature and International Nursing Index (INI).

Contributors

CONSULTING EDITOR

STEPHEN D. KRAU, PhD, RN, CNE
Associate Professor, Vanderbilt University School of Nursing, Nashville, Tennessee

EDITORS

JENNIFER KIM, DNP, GNP-BC, FNAP
Assistant Professor of Nursing, Vanderbilt University School of Nursing, Nashville, Tennessee

SALLY MILLER, PhD, RN
Assistant Professor of Nursing, Vanderbilt University School of Nursing, Nashville, Tennessee

AUTHORS

NATALIE R. BAKER, DNP, ANP-BC, GNP-BC
Assistant Professor, University of Alabama at Birmingham School of Nursing, Birmingham, Alabama

KALA K. BLAKELY, DNP, NP-C
Assistant Professor, University of Alabama at Birmingham School of Nursing, Birmingham, Alabama

EILEEN R. CHASENS, PhD, RN, FAAN
Associate Professor, Department of Health and Community Systems, University of Pittsburgh School of Nursing, Pittsburgh, Pennsylvania

NEVA L. CROGAN, PhD, ARNP, GNP-BC, ACHPN, FNGNA, FAAN
Professor, Department of Nursing, Gonzaga University, Spokane, Washington

GRACE E. DEAN, PhD, RN
Associate Professor, Department of Biobehavioral Health and Clinical Sciences, University at Buffalo School of Nursing, Buffalo, New York

DEANNA GRAY-MICELI, PhD, GNP-BC, FAAN, FAANP, FGSA, FNAP
Assistant Professor, Rutgers University School of Nursing, Newark, New Jersey; Claire M. Fagin Post-Doctoral Fellow (2002-2004), Associate, Institute for Health, Health Care Policy and Aging Research, New Brunswick, New Jersey

MELODEE HARRIS, PhD, APRN, GNP-BC
University of Arkansas for Medical Sciences, College of Nursing, Little Rock, Arkansas

ANN L. HORGAS, RN, PhD, FGSA, FAAN
Associate Professor, Department of Biobehavioral Nursing Science, University of Florida
College of Nursing, Gainesville, Florida

JENNIFER KIM, DNP, GNP-BC, FNAP
Assistant Professor of Nursing, Vanderbilt University School of Nursing, Nashville,
Tennessee

CATHY A. MAXWELL, PhD, RN
Vanderbilt University School of Nursing, Nashville, Tennessee

MARTHA JANE MOHLER, NP-C, MPH, PhD
Professor, Arizona Center on Aging, Division of Geriatrics, General Internal Medicine,
and Palliative Medicine, College of Medicine, Mel and Enid Zuckerman College of Public
Health, University of Arizona, Tucson, Arizona

JONNA L. MORRIS, BSN, RN
PhD Student, Department of Health and Community Systems, University of Pittsburgh
School of Nursing, Pittsburgh, Pennsylvania

ROSE W. MURPHREE, DNP, MSN, RN, CWOCN, CFCN
Assistant Clinical Professor, Emory University, Nell Hodgson Woodruff School of Nursing,
Director, Wound, Ostomy, and Continence Nursing Education Center, Atlanta, Georgia

ABBY LUCK PARISH, DNP, ANP-BC, GNP-BC, FNAP
Vanderbilt University School of Nursing, Nashville, Tennessee

RACHEL PETERSON, MA, MPH
Senior Health Educator, Arizona Center on Aging, University of Arizona College of
Medicine, Tucson, Arizona

JESSICA A.R. SEARCY, DNP, FNP-BC, WHNP-BC
Instructor of Nursing, Women's Health Nurse Practitioner Program, Vanderbilt University
School of Nursing, Nashville, Tennessee

RUTH E. TAYLOR-PILIAE, PhD, RN, FAHA
Associate Professor, University of Arizona College of Nursing, Tucson, Arizona

JINJIAO WANG, PhD, RN
Vanderbilt University School of Nursing, Nashville, Tennessee

CARLEARA WEISS, PhD, RN
Department of Biobehavioral Health and Clinical Sciences, University at Buffalo School of
Nursing, Buffalo, New York

Contents

> Frailty is a public health crisis for an aging society. As a concept and condition, frailty is poorly understood and underrecognized in clinical settings. Nurses play an important role as frontline providers who care for aging adults. The aim of this article is to raise awareness among nurses about frailty and to discuss the recognition and management of this prevailing condition. The authors present conceptual definitions and models of frailty, a brief discussion of the underlying biological mechanisms and evidence-based interventions for frailty identification, and approaches to delay and decrease the burden of frailty.

> Cognitive decline in older persons can be pathologic or occur as a part of the normal aging process. Delirium, depression, and dementia are geriatric syndromes and neurocognitive disorders that are the result of cognitive decline associated with pathology. This overview is a brief guide on cognitive decline and how to identify, manage, and treat associated neurocognitive disorders, including delirium, depression, and dementia.

> Pain is a common experience for many older adults. Significant efforts have been undertaken to address and improve the assessment of pain in older adults over the past 2 decades. There have been many empirical studies and several expert panel statements to guide health care providers in the best practices for assessing pain in this population. This article provides a conceptual model that summarizes causes and consequences of pain and highlights the relationship between acute and persistent pain. Recommendations for pain assessment tools, including those developed for use in cognitively impaired elders, are presented.

> Impaired sleep increases in prevalence in older adults, with multiple possible causes that can interact with each other and can lead to poor health outcomes. This article describes normal changes in sleep with aging, sleep disorders that increase in prevalence in older adults, medications and sleep, and medical conditions and psychosocial conditions

associated with impaired sleep. In addition, a brief assessment that nurses could use to assess for impaired sleep and nonpharmacologic interventions to improve sleep are discussed.

Altered skin integrity increases the chance of infection, impaired mobility, and decreased function and may result in the loss of limb or, sometimes, life. Skin is affected by both intrinsic and extrinsic factors. Intrinsic factors can include altered nutritional status, vascular disease issues, and diabetes. Extrinsic factors include falls, accidents, pressure, immobility, and surgical procedures. Ensuring skin integrity in the elderly requires a team approach and includes the individual, caregivers, and clinicians. The twenty-first century clinician has several online, evidence-based tools to assist with optimal treatment plans. Understanding best practices in addressing skin integrity issues can promote positive outcomes with the elderly.

Gastrointestinal (GI) age-related changes create alterations in the body's ability to digest, absorb, and excrete nutrients, medications, and alcohol and disrupts GI immunity responses. All older adults exhibit some degree of swallowing difficulty, also known as senescent swallowing. The effects of chronic disease and sustained use of alcohol, tobacco, and medications often exacerbate age-related GI dysfunction. Older adults often have nonspecific complaints, warranting a thorough health history and physical examination, including prescription and over-the-counter medications. Colorectal cancer screening tests should be discussed with all older adults because of the high incidence of colorectal cancer in this patient population.

Nutritional problems, such as malnutrition, dehydration, and electrolyte imbalance, are multifaceted and complex issues for older adults. This article describes these potential nutritional problems and then discusses evidence-based assessment strategies and treatment modalities that target these problems. Micronutrient deficiency is explored and evidence-based supplementation discussed. Many factors contribute to weight loss and malnutrition in older adults. These factors are classified as social, psychological, and/or biological. Addressing these issues and the influence of oral health on food intake are imperative to enhancing the overall quality of life for older adults.

Urinary incontinence (UI) is an international problem, affecting a high percentage of geriatric women. Nurses caring for geriatric women of all ages should be aware of the problem of UI and familiarize themselves with the potential treatment options for these patients. This article focuses on the prevalence, burden, clinical application, and management recommendations for the different types of UI.

Polypharmacy in older adults is a global problem that has recently worsened. Approximately 30% of adults aged 65 years and older in developed countries take 5 or more medications. Although prescribed and over-the-counter medications may improve a wide range of health problems, they also may cause or contribute to harm, especially in older adults. Polypharmacy in older adults is associated with worsening of geriatric syndromes and adverse drug events. Given the risks and burdens of polypharmacy and potentially inappropriate medications, nurses must use patient-centered approaches and nonpharmacologic strategies to treat common symptoms and to optimize patient function and quality of life.

The Centers for Medicare and Medicaid services report nearly 55% of Medicare beneficiaries older than 85 experience impaired mobility and nearly 28% (n = 671,833) of these individuals have difficulty getting help. Impaired mobility is a precursor to disability, which has notable clinical significance and importance to older adults. Using case exemplars of older adults who have experienced a "serious" fall, along with evidence-based research, the physical, psychosocial, emotional, and clinical consequences are discussed, along with assessment parameters and interventions for maximizing function and early mobility.

Falls in older adults are the result of several risk factors across biological and behavioral aspects of the person, along with environmental factors. Falls can trigger a downward spiral in activities of daily living, independence, and overall health outcomes. Clinicians who care for older adults should screen them annually for falls. A multifactorial comprehensive clinical fall assessment coupled with tailored interventions can result in a dramatic public health impact, while improving older adult quality of life. For community-dwelling older adults, effective fall prevention has the potential to reduce serious fall-related injuries, emergency room visits, hospitalizations, institutionalization, and functional decline.

NURSING CLINICS OF NORTH AMERICA

Preface

Geriatric Syndromes: Meeting a Growing Challenge

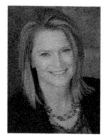
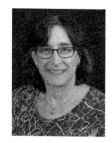

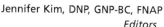

Jennifer Kim, DNP, GNP-BC, FNAP   Sally Miller, PhD, RN
Editors

The world is aging. The older adult population is growing rapidly in the United States and worldwide. It is estimated that older adults will represent 20% of the US population by 2030, at which time they will exceed the number of the young for the first time in history.[1] Given advancements in medical care, life expectancy in this country is increasing. Current life expectancy at birth is 78.8 years.[2] Those who survive to age 65 can be expected to live, on average, until age 84, and those who survive to age 85 are expected to live to age 91.[2] "Old-old" adults, those aged ≥85, is the fastest growing age group in the United States and will represent 4.5% of American population by 2030.[3] Old-old adults have more health conditions than their younger counterparts. Along with a growing percentage of older adults is a growing public concern about the ability to adequately care for their unique and complex physical and psychosocial needs. Normal changes of aging combined with accrued diseases and conditions increase an older adult's vulnerability. More than two-thirds of all Medicare beneficiaries have two or more chronic conditions, and more than 15% have six or more.[4] The occurrence of at least one chronic medical condition is associated with the presence of at least one geriatric syndrome.[5]

Geriatric syndromes are clinical conditions commonly found in older adults and are associated with increased morbidity and mortality. They share underlying contributing factors and involve multiple organ systems, but they do not fit into specific disease categories.[6] Common geriatric syndromes include urinary incontinence, cognitive impairment, delirium, falls, pressure ulcers, polypharmacy, and weight loss. Geriatric syndromes contribute to poor health outcomes, including disability, institutionalization, and dependence.[6]

In their various clinical roles, nurses have the opportunity to identify geriatric syndromes through screening and thorough assessments. Furthermore, nurses are in a position to refer to, and collaborate with, appropriate disciplines, family, and

Nurs Clin N Am 52 (2017) ix–x
http://dx.doi.org/10.1016/j.cnur.2017.06.001
0029-6465/17/© 2017 Published by Elsevier Inc.   nursing.theclinics.com

community resources to implement patient-centered interventions. Articles in this issue address the importance of early identification of geriatric syndromes and include key information regarding appropriate screening measures, in-depth assessment strategies, nursing interventions, and collaborative care.

We hope this issue will provide vital information for nurses across the health care continuum as together we face the challenge of providing care for the complex needs of older adults at risk for or experiencing geriatric syndromes.

Jennifer Kim, DNP, GNP-BC, FNAP
Vanderbilt University School of Nursing
461 21st Avenue South
Nashville, TN 37240, USA

Sally Miller, PhD, RN
Vanderbilt University School of Nursing
461 21st Avenue South
Nashville, TN 37240, USA

E-mail addresses:
jennifer.kim@vanderbilt.edu (J. Kim)
sally.m.miller@vanderbilt.edu (S. Miller)

REFERENCES

1. Centers for Disease Control and Prevention. The state of aging and health in America 2013. Atlanta (GA): Centers for Disease Control and Prevention, US Department of Health and Human Services; 2013.
2. National Vital Statistics Report. 2017. Available at: https://www.cdc.gov/nchs/data/nvsr/nvsr66/nvsr66_03.pdf. Accessed May 2017.
3. U.S. Census Bureau. 2010. Available at: https://www.census.gov/prod/2014pubs/p25-1140.pdf. Accessed May 2017.
4. Lochner KA, Shoff CM. County-level variation in prevalence of multiple chronic conditions among Medicare beneficiaries, 2012. Prev Chronic Dis 2015;12:E07.
5. Lee PG, Cigolle C, Blaum C. The co-occurrence of chronic diseases and geriatric syndromes: the health and retirement study. J Am Geriatr Soc 2009;57(3):511–6.
6. Inouye SK, Studenski S, Tinetti ME, et al. Geriatric syndromes: clinical, research, and policy implications of a core geriatric concept. J Am Geriatr Soc 2007; 55(5):780–91.

Understanding Frailty
A Nurse's Guide

Cathy A. Maxwell, PhD, RN*, Jinjiao Wang, PhD, RN

KEYWORDS

- Frailty • Older adults • Models of frailty • Mechanisms of frailty • Frailty interventions

KEY POINTS

- Frailty is a public health crisis of population aging.
- Models of frailty include the frailty phenotype and the cumulative deficit model.
- Frailty is a superior predictor of poor outcomes over age and comorbidities.
- Standardized frailty screening should occur in all clinical settings.
- Physical activity is the overarching intervention for prevention and management of frailty.

Frailty is an overarching public health crisis of population aging; however, as a concept and condition, frailty is poorly understood and underrecognized in clinical settings. Frailty represents the effect of age-related decline in multiple physiologic systems and leads to vulnerability to stressors, disability, and death. Physiologic dysregulation that contributes to the trajectory of frailty often begins in midlife before clinical manifestations are apparent. In fact, the intermediate stage known as pre-frailty is related to early functional decline that can be detected and intervened upon to delay development of advanced frailty and disability.[1,2] Nurses play an important role as frontline providers who care for aging adults. The aim of this article is to raise awareness about frailty among nurses and to discuss recognition and management of this prevailing condition. The authors present conceptual definitions and models of frailty, a brief discussion of underlying biological mechanisms, and evidence-based interventions to consider in clinical settings that care for older adults.

DEFINING FRAILTY

Broadly, frailty is defined as a clinically recognizable state of increasing vulnerability resulting from aging associated decline in reserve and function across multiple physiologic systems, thus, compromising the ability to recover from endogenous and

The authors have no disclosures or financial conflicts of interest.
Vanderbilt University School of Nursing, 461 21st Avenue South, Nashville, TN 37240, USA
* Corresponding author.
E-mail address: Cathy.maxwell@vanderbilt.edu

exogenous stressors.[3] The occurrence of stressors (ie, illness, injury, psychosocial stress) exacerbates functional decline among frail individuals and places them at higher risk for negative health-related outcomes. The development of frailty is a novel perspective to health and wellness that gained considerable attention over the past several years as a stronger indicator than chronologic aging of biological aging and survival.[4–6] Ensuing frailty is characterized by gradual loss of energy, strength, endurance, and motor control (eg, grip strength, gait speed, balance) (**Fig. 1**). Coupled with loss of integrity of the axial skeleton (osteoporosis, vertebral deterioration, stress fractures), frailty leads to falls with injury, further decline, and death.

MODELS OF FRAILTY

Two models of frailty are predominant in scientific research and clinical application. The *Fried phenotype model of frailty*, derived from the Cardiovascular Health Study,[7] identified 5 criteria/characteristics that define frailty from a physical perspective that include weight loss, self-reported exhaustion, low physical activity (energy expenditure), slow gait speed, and weakness (grip strength) (**Table 1**).

A second model derived from the Canadian Study of Health and Aging is *the Rockwood cumulative deficit model or frailty index*.[8–10] The original model identified 70 deficits (symptoms, signs, laboratory values, disabilities) that occur as frailty develops (**Box 1**). Modified versions of the frailty index contain lower numbers of variables ranging from 12 to 40 from the original 70.[11–14] A frailty index is created by dividing the total number of deficits by the number of variables examined. The Rockwood model lends itself to a more holistic view of frailty; however, critics argue that this perspective is a more difficult concept to operationalize.[4,15]

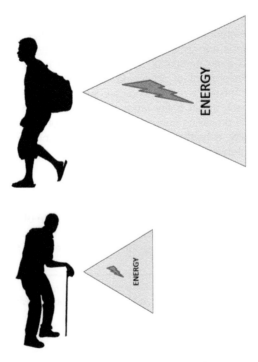

Fig. 1. Frailty: gradual loss of energy, strength, endurance, and motor control.

Table 1	
Fried phenotype criteria and measurement indices	
FP Criteria	**Measurement**
Weakness	Grip strength <20th percentile
Slowness	Walking time (15 feet): slowest 20% by sex and height
Low level of physical activity	Bottom 20th percentile of calculated kcal as measured by the Minnesota Leisure Time Activity Questionnaire
Exhaustion	Self-reported, based on items in the Center for Epidemiologic Studies Depression Scale
Weight loss	>10% of unintentional weight loss during the prior year

From Fried LP, Tangen CM, Walston J, et al. Frailty in older adults: evidence for a phenotype. J Gerontol A Biol Sci Med Sci 2001;56(3):M146–56.

Both models are predictive of frailty and useful for frailty identification; however, clinical application is often based on usability and practical considerations. The Fried phenotype model is more commonly used for screening purposes, whereas the Rockwood frailty index provides a more precise method of quantifying frailty and discriminating between levels of frailty.[16,17]

Andrew Clegg[18,19] proposed another frailty phenotype based on the cumulative deficit model that includes 5 components: sarcopenia, anorexia, fatigue, risk of fall, and poor physical health. This perspective posits that the 5 components emerge as individuals experience chronic disease and deconditioning. A theoretic line of decompensation is reached when a minor stressor (eg, urinary tract infection, minor fall) leads to a disproportionate change from independence to dependence (**Fig. 2**).

Subcategories of Frailty

In 2013, a consensus conference on frailty[4] defined a subcategory of frailty, that is, *physical frailty*, and noted 4 important points that distinguish physical frailty as a distinct entity. Physical frailty is based on the Fried phenotype and is defined as "a medical syndrome with multiple causes and contributors that is characterized by diminished strength, endurance, and reduced physiologic function that increases an individual's vulnerability for developing increased dependency and/or death."[4] Experts also note the following: (1) not all disabled persons are frail, but frailty can lead to disability; (2) frailty differs from sarcopenia (muscle wasting) and is a more multifaceted concept; (3) diagnosis of frailty should be determined by a geriatrician using criteria of well-defined models; and (4) physical frailty differs from multimorbidity in that comorbidities are more pervasive and occur in 3 of 4 persons greater than the age of 65.[4]

Another subcategory of frailty is *cognitive frailty*, defined as the simultaneous presence of both physical frailty and cognitive impairment, excluding concurrent Alzheimer dementia or other dementias.[20] Recent research suggests a prolonged preclinical phase of ensuing physical frailty before the onset of dementia symptoms. A systematic review revealed that physical frailty constructs (eg, weakness, slowness, low physical activity) were linked to late-life cognitive impairment due to underlying mechanisms that are linked to vascular, inflammatory, nutritional, and metabolic influences.[21] Evidence suggests that cognitive frailty may be reversible with nutritional, physical, or cognitive interventions, singly or in combination.[22]

Box 1
Cumulative deficits for frailty index

Cumulative deficits (70 variables from the Canadian Study of Health and Aging)

- Changes in everyday activities
- Head and neck problems
- Poor muscle tone in neck
- Bradykinesia, facial
- Problems getting dressed
- Problems with bathing
- Problems carrying out personal grooming
- Urinary incontinence
- Toileting problems
- Bulk difficulties
- Rectal problems
- Gastrointestinal problems
- Problems cooking
- Sucking problems
- Problems going out alone
- Impaired mobility
- Musculoskeletal problems
- Bradykinesia of the limbs
- Poor muscle tone in limbs
- Poor limb coordination
- Poor coordination, trunk
- Poor standing posture
- Irregular gait pattern
- Falls
- Mood problems
- Feeling sad, blue, depressed
- History of depressed mood
- Tiredness all the time
- Depression (clinical impression)
- Sleep changes
- Restlessness
- Memory changes
- Short-term memory impairment
- Long-term memory impairment
- Changes in general mental functioning
- Onset of cognitive symptoms
- Clouding or delirium

- Paranoid features
- History relevant to cognitive impairment or loss
- Family history relevant to cognitive impairment or loss
- Impaired vibration
- Tremor at rest
- Postural tremor
- Intention tremor
- History of Parkinson disease
- Family history of degenerative disease
- Seizures, partial complex
- Seizure, generalized
- Syncope or blackouts
- Headache
- Cerebrovascular problems
- History of stroke
- History of diabetes mellitus
- Arterial hypertension
- Peripheral pulses
- Cardiac problems
- Myocardial infarction
- Arrhythmia
- Congestive heart failure
- Lung problems
- Respiratory problems
- History of thyroid disease
- Thyroid problems
- Skin problems
- Malignant disease
- Breast problems
- Abdominal problems
- Presence of snout reflex
- Presence of palmomental reflex
- Other medical history

From Mitnitski AB, Mogilner AJ, Rockwood K. Accumulation of deficits as a proxy measure of aging. ScientificWorldJournal 2001;1:323–36.

Conceptual Perspectives on Frailty

A PubMed search on "frailty as a concept" produces more than 200 articles with 28 having keywords "frailty" and "concept" in the title. Frailty scholars have published perspectives that are based on the 2 prevailing models of frailty (phenotype, deficit

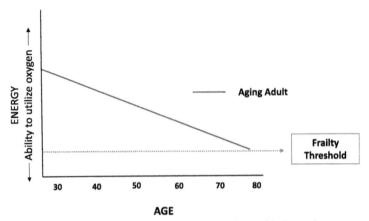

Fig. 2. Line of decompensation: minor stressor leads to loss of independence.

accumulation) and other perspectives that complement the phenotype and deficit accumulation models.

In 1993, Walter M. Bortz, MD[23] published an article in the *Journal of the American Geriatric Society* titled, "The Physics of Frailty." This work is an interesting perspective that links frailty to the physical sciences (biology, physics, chemistry) by suggesting that frailty may be driven by the molecular forces of nature (eg, thermodynamics, energetics). Emerging evidence that links frailty with poor health outcomes supports this perspective (see next section, Predictors of outcomes).[24,25] Bortz[26] highlights the effect of use and disuse (movement, exercise) on form (posture) and function (strength, endurance, balance). A subsequent publication focuses on altered energy loads and proposes that frailty is a body-wide set of deteriorations in multiple systems that have a common final pathway linked to decline in physical activity.

Another expert and geriatrician, John E. Morley, MD, is a prolific writer with more than 300 publications related to aging and many articles focused on frailty. In 2002, an editorial, titled "Something About Frailty," proposed 4 major intrinsic pathways that lead to frailty, including sarcopenia (muscle wasting), metabolic alterations (ie, hormonal changes, increased cytokines), atherosclerosis, and malnutrition.[27] In addition to physiologic mechanisms, these factors are impacted by socioeconomic factors (low income, low education, lack of social support). More recently, Morley focused on the pathogenesis of sarcopenia in a publication entitled, *Frailty and Sarcopenia: The New Geriatric Giants.*[5]

FRAILTY AS A PREDICTOR OF POOR OUTCOMES

As frailty emerged as a public health priority, the number of studies linking frailty to health outcomes has proliferated. Systematic reviews published over the past 2 years examine the influence of frailty on multiple outcomes in various older populations, including all patients,[28] postoperative surgical patients,[29] medical patients,[30] cardiac surgical procedures,[31] and patients with cancer.[32] Studies overwhelmingly indicate that frailty is the predominant predictor of poor outcomes, including in-hospital mortality, 1-year mortality, hospitalization, disability, falls, adverse clinical outcomes, hospital length of stay, discharge disposition, functional decline, and treatment complications.[28–32] Studies note the superiority of frailty over chronologic age, comorbidities, race, and sex and highlight the importance frailty in risk identification.[7,33–36]

Underlying physiologic mechanisms leading to frailty and poor health outcomes have been increasingly explored in recent years with recognized overlaps among mechanisms. Although this article does not address mechanisms of frailty, the predominant pathways deserve mention: brain pathways (eg, loss of neurons and neuroplasticity),[37] endocrine/hormonal (eg, decrease and dysregulation),[38] immune (senescence),[39,40] inflammation (eg, hypersensitivity to stimuli),[41] metabolic (eg, altered enzyme and glycation processes),[42] and oxidative stress (eg, proliferation of free radicals).[43]

A novel pathway that may help to explain these causative mechanisms at the cellular level relates to mitochondria, that is, energy production. Mitochondria is the organelle that controls processes of cellular respiration and energy production, and also the only organelle (excluding the nucleus) that contains its own genetic material (mitochondrial DNA [mtDNA]), which encodes molecular elements necessary for electron transport and cellular respiration. Mitochondrial research is on the increase among medical sciences with increasing recognition that mitochondria exert systemic effects by altering complex physiologic functions. Specifically, decreased mtDNA copy number (indicating decreased mitochondrial activity) is associated with poor outcomes, including all-cause mortality,[44] malignant processes,[45] chronic kidney disease,[46] and heart failure.[47] Future research that explores these links may shed further light on mechanisms of frailty.

APPLICATION OF FRAILTY RESEARCH IN CLINICAL SETTINGS

In light of the preponderance of evidence that supports the link between frailty and poor clinical outcomes, this section describes evidence-based interventions for identification (screening) and delaying and decreasing the burden of frailty (management). A comprehensive geriatric assessment is foundational to clinical management of frailty and constitutes the gold standard for care of frail older adults.[48]

Screening and Risk Identification

Identification of frailty in older adults begins with established screening processes. Multiple reviews advocate for standardized frailty screening in clinical settings[3,49–52] with consideration of capabilities within clinical settings (ie, time, ease of use, personnel) and abilities of older populations. For example, in acute care settings, older adults are often in pain, sedated, or unable to undergo physical testing; self-report or proxy-report instruments may be the most appropriate method of assessment. Primary care settings may be more appropriate for screening procedures that entail performance of physical tests (ie, walking speed, handgrip).

A wide array of frailty screening instruments is available for clinicians. A recent review of frailty measurement instruments provides an overview of 29 measurements and compares them according to model of frailty, time to administer, number of items, components, scoring, requirement of measurement, and applicable setting.[53] **Table 2** provides a list of commonly used screening instruments in clinical settings, along with a brief description of content. When choosing the appropriate instrument for frailty screening, Clegg and colleagues[19] recommended clinicians consider the following features: (1) predictive of poor outcomes, (2) predictive of response to specific therapies, (3) supported by biological causative theory, and (4) simplicity of use. Regardless of the screening instrument used, the priority is identification so that management strategies can be implemented in early stages of the frailty trajectory.

Table 2 Commonly used frailty screening instruments	
Instrument	**Description of Content**
Edmonton Frailty Scale[54]	11 items in 9 domains (cognition, general health, functional independence, social support, medication use, nutrition, mood, continence, functional performance) scored from 0 to 2
Tilburg Frailty Indicator[55]	25 items; demographic data; domains: physical, psychological, and social components of frailty
PRISMA-7[56]	7 items, yes/no format; domains: age, sex, health limitations (2), need for assistance (2), use of assistive devices
Groningen Frailty Indicator[57]	15 items, yes/no format; domains: mobility, vision, hearing, nutrition, comorbidity, cognition, psychosocial, physical fitness
Sherbrooke Postal Questionnaire[58]	6 items; functional autonomy (ADLs, mobility, communication, cognition, IADLs)
Vulnerable Elders Survey[59]	13 items; domains: age, self-rated health, common physical activities, ADLs
Identification of Seniors at Risk[60]	6 items, yes/no format; domains: need for assistance, past hospitalizations, vision, memory, number of medications
Hospital Admission Risk Profile[61]	3 domains: age, IADLs, cognition (abbreviated MMSE); score range: 0–5
Short Physical Performance Battery[62]	3 domains: balance, gait speed, chair stand
Rapid screening tools	
FRAIL Questionnaire[63]	5 items, yes/no format; fatigue, resistance, ambulation, illnesses, loss of weight
Clinical Frailty Scale[8]	9 point scale from very fit (1) to terminally ill (9); silhouettes and descriptions
Gérontopôle Frailty Screening Tool[64]	6 items, yes/no format; living arrangements, weight loss, fatigue, mobility, memory loss, gait speed

Abbreviations: ADLs, activities of daily living; IADLs, instrumental activities of daily living; MMSE, Mini-Mental State Examination.

Interventions for Frailty

An understanding of best clinical management strategies to address frailty in multiple settings is evolving. Detailed evidence from high-quality studies is lacking[65,66]; however, new studies and systematic reviews are underway.[67,68] This article reports on currently available evidence on frailty interventions.

Physical activity is the overarching intervention for prevention and management of frailty. Existing systematic reviews support the value of exercise interventions.[69,70] Interventions most effective in decreasing falls and improving gait ability are multicomponent in format and address multiple domains of strength, endurance, and balance as opposed to single domains. Such interventions should be repeated at least 3 times per week for 30 to 45 minutes and sustained for more than 5 months.[70,71] These recommendations are supported by the World Health Organization[72] and other leading senior care organizations, including the National Council on Aging (https://www.ncoa.org/), the National Institute on Aging (https://go4life.nia.nih.gov/), and the American Association of Retired Persons (http://www.aarp.org/health/healthy-living/). An example of an individually designed intervention for prevention of frailty might include an exercise routine with free weights (strength), brisk walking (endurance), and yoga or tai chi (balance). For an older adult who is already frail, the intervention can be modified to include the use of resistance bands (strength), walking to tolerance (endurance), and chair yoga/tai chi. Engagement in exercise that is fun and enjoyable and that promotes social interaction increases the likelihood of continued participation[73]; thus, discussions with patients should elicit feedback about preferences. For example, walking is the most popular leisure-time physical activity in older adults and has lower risk for injury compared with other modes of exercise such as jogging.[74]

Biologic theories of frailty explain benefits of exercise and increased physical activity. Although reduced in older adults, studies show that resistance training increases muscle mass and strength and increases free fat mass loss.[75,76] Exercise promotes anti-inflammatory and antioxidative stress effects that slow muscle wasting and increase protein synthesis,[77] and all of these are underlying mechanisms of frailty. In addition, from the cellular aging perspective, because frailty represents vulnerability to stressors, preservation of systems that control cellular responses to stress is a strategy for addressing the frailty phenotype.

Along with physical activity as the primary intervention for frailty, other considerations are important in the care of vulnerable elders. An integrative review of supportive care approaches for frailty in acute settings identified priorities.[78] Hospitalization of frail older adults is an emotionally and physically stressful event for patients and families because it often highlights functional decline and approaching end of life.[79] Nurses and other clinicians can facilitate understanding regarding the frailty trajectory by providing prognostic information and helping families understand what to expect in terms of gradual decline in function. Communication is crucial as providers connect and engage in ways that promote shared decision making. Nicholson and colleagues[78] support the theme of *building a picture of the individual person and circumstances* to facilitate communication. For example, the nurse might ask a patient and family to describe the patient's physical abilities and limitations over the prior 3 years. The nurse could follow up with the use of information and pictographs to explain gradual loss of strength and endurance associated with frailty. Consistency of communication and support through transitions of care is also important because many frail patients transfer to post–acute care facilities after hospital discharge.

SUMMARY

The objective of this article was to raise awareness of frailty for nurses who provide care to older adults in a variety of clinical settings by providing a thorough overview about frailty that might serve as a guide for clinical care. A simple and complementary description is that *frailty represents a gradual loss of the human body's ability to generate energy to sustain itself*. This process will eventually occur in most of us. Our aim is to advance understanding among patients, families, providers, and the public in hopes of broader dialogue to optimize living as we experience the changes and challenges associated with aging. In light of nurses' natural advantage at patient education, providing communication about frailty to older patients can facilitate understanding about frailty as a condition and actions to delay onset and lower the burden of frailty.

REFERENCES

1. Fernández-Garrido J, Ruiz-Ros V, Buigues C, et al. Clinical features of prefrail older individuals and emerging peripheral biomarkers: a systematic review. Arch Gerontol Geriatr 2014;59(1):7–17.

2. Acosta-Benito MA, Sevilla-Machuca I. Using prefrailty to detect early disability. J Fam Community Med 2016;23(3):140.
3. Xue QL. The frailty syndrome: definition and natural history. Clin Geriatr Med 2011;27(1):1–15.
4. Morley JE, Vellas B, Abellan van Kan G, et al. Frailty consensus: a call to action. J Am Med Dir Assoc 2013;14(6):392–7.
5. Morley JE. Frailty and sarcopenia: the new geriatric giants. Rev Invest Clin 2015; 68(2):59–67.
6. Shamliyan T, Talley KM, Ramakrishnan R, et al. Association of frailty with survival: a systematic literature review. Ageing Res Rev 2013;12(2):719–36.
7. Fried LP, Tangen CM, Walston J, et al. Frailty in older adults: evidence for a phenotype. J Gerontol A Biol Sci Med Sci 2001;56(3):M146–56.
8. Rockwood K, Song X, MacKnight C, et al. A global clinical measure of fitness and frailty in elderly people. Can Med Assoc J 2005;173(5):489–95.
9. Rockwood K, Mitnitski A. Frailty in relation to the accumulation of deficits. J Gerontol A Biol Sci Med Sci 2007;62(7):722–7.
10. Mitnitski AB, Mogilner AJ, Rockwood K. Accumulation of deficits as a proxy measure of aging. ScientificWorldJournal 2001;1:323–36.
11. Mitnitski AB, Song X, Rockwood K. The estimation of relative fitness and frailty in community-dwelling older adults using self-report data. J Gerontol A Biol Sci Med Sci 2004;59(6):M627–32.
12. Yu P, Song X, Shi J, et al. Frailty and survival of older Chinese adults in urban and rural areas: results from the Beijing longitudinal study of aging. Arch Gerontol Geriatr 2012;54(1):3–8.
13. Adams P, Ghanem T, Stachler R, et al. Frailty as a predictor of morbidity and mortality in inpatient head and neck surgery. JAMA Otolaryngol Head Neck Surg 2013;139(8):783–9.
14. Hoogendijk EO, Theou O, Rockwood K, et al. Development and validation of a frailty index in the Longitudinal Aging Study Amsterdam. Aging Clin Exp Res 2016;1–7.
15. Boers M, Jentoft AJC. A new concept of health can improve the definition of frailty. Calcif Tissue Int 2015;97(5):429–31.
16. Malmstrom TK, Miller DK, Morley JE. A comparison of four frailty models. J Am Geriatr Soc 2014;62(4):721–6.
17. Cigolle CT, Ofstedal MB, Tian Z, et al. Comparing models of frailty: the health and retirement study. J Am Geriatr Soc 2009;57(5):830–9.
18. Clegg A, Young J. The frailty syndrome. Clin Med (Lond) 2011;11(1):72–5.
19. Clegg A, Young J, Iliffe S, et al. Frailty in elderly people. Lancet 2013;381(9868): 752–62.
20. Kelaiditi E, Cesari M, Canevelli M, et al. Cognitive frailty: rational and definition from an (IANA/IAGG) international consensus group. J Nutr Health Aging 2013; 17(9):726–34.
21. Panza F, Solfrizzi V, Barulli MR, et al. Cognitive frailty: a systematic review of epidemiological and neurobiological evidence of an age-related clinical condition. Rejuvenation Res 2015;18(5):389–412.
22. Ng TP, Feng L, Nyunt MSZ, et al. Nutritional, physical, cognitive, and combination interventions and frailty reversal among older adults: a randomized controlled trial. Am J Med 2015;128(11):1225–36.e1.
23. Bortz WM. The physics of frailty. J Am Geriatr Soc 1993;41(9):1004–8.
24. Landi F, Abbatecola AM, Provinciali M, et al. Moving against frailty: does physical activity matter? Biogerontology 2010;11(5):537–45.

25. Hepple RT. Mitochondrial involvement and impact in aging skeletal muscle. Front Aging Neurosci 2014;6:211.
26. Bortz WM. A conceptual framework of frailty a review. J Gerontol A Biol Sci Med Sci 2002;57(5):M283–8.
27. Morley JE, Perry HM, Miller DK. Editorial: something about frailty. J Gerontol A Biol Sci Med Sci 2002;57(11):M698–704.
28. Vermeiren S, Vella-Azzopardi R, Beckwée D, et al. Frailty and the prediction of negative health outcomes: a meta-analysis. J Am Med Dir Assoc 2016;17(12):1163.e1-17.
29. Oakland K, Nadler R, Cresswell L, et al. Systematic review and meta-analysis of the association between frailty and outcome in surgical patients. Ann R Coll Surg Engl 2016;98(2):80–5.
30. Ritt M, Gaßmann KG, Sieber CC. Significance of frailty for predicting adverse clinical outcomes in different patient groups with specific medical conditions. Z Gerontol Geriatr 2016;49(7):567–72.
31. Kim DH, Kim CA, Placide S, et al. Preoperative frailty assessment and outcomes at 6 months or later in older adults undergoing cardiac surgical procedures: a systematic review. Ann Intern Med 2016;165(9):650–60.
32. Handforth C, Clegg A, Young C, et al. The prevalence and outcomes of frailty in older cancer patients: a systematic review. Ann Oncol 2015;26(6):1091–101.
33. Joseph B, Pandit V, Zangbar B, et al. Superiority of frailty over age in predicting outcomes among geriatric trauma patients: a prospective analysis. JAMA Surg 2014;149(8):766–72.
34. Maxwell CA, Mion LC, Mukherjee K, et al. Preinjury physical frailty and cognitive impairment among geriatric trauma patients determine postinjury functional recovery and survival. J Trauma Acute Care Surg 2016;80(2):195–203.
35. Ommundsen N, Wyller TB, Nesbakken A, et al. Frailty is an independent predictor of survival in older patients with colorectal cancer. Oncologist 2014;19(12):1268–75.
36. Ravaglia G, Forti P, Lucicesare A, et al. Development of an easy prognostic score for frailty outcomes in the aged. Age Ageing 2008;37(2):161–6.
37. Buchman AS, Yu L, Wilson RS, et al. Association of brain pathology with the progression of frailty in older adults. Neurology 2013;80(22):2055–61.
38. Bishop NA, Lu T, Yankner BA. Neural mechanisms of ageing and cognitive decline. Nature 2010;464(7288):529–35.
39. Leng SX, Hung W, Cappola AR, et al. White blood cell counts, insulinlike growth factor-1 levels, and frailty in community-dwelling older women. J Gerontol A Biol Sci Med Sci 2009;64(4):499–502.
40. Leng SX, Xue QL, Tian J, et al. Inflammation and frailty in older women. J Am Geriatr Soc 2007;55(6):864–71.
41. Zhu Y, Liu Z, Wang Y, et al. C-reactive protein, frailty and overnight hospital admission in elderly individuals: a population-based study. Arch Gerontol Geriatr 2016;64:1–5.
42. Corona G, Polesel J, Fratino L, et al. Metabolomics biomarkers of frailty in elderly breast cancer patients. J Cell Physiol 2014;229(7):898–902.
43. Harman D. Aging: a theory based on free radical and radiation chemistry. J Gerontol 1956;11(3):298–300.
44. Ashar FN, Moes A, Moore AZ, et al. Association of mitochondrial DNA levels with frailty and all-cause mortality. J Mol Med 2015;93(2):177–86.

45. van Osch FH, Voets AM, Schouten LJ, et al. Mitochondrial DNA copy number in colorectal cancer: between tissue comparisons, clinicopathological characteristics and survival. Carcinogenesis 2015;36(12):1502–10.

46. Tin A, Grams ME, Ashar FN, et al. Association between mitochondrial DNA copy number in peripheral blood and incident CKD in the atherosclerosis risk in communities study. J Am Soc Nephrol 2016;27(8):2467–73.

47. Huang J, Tan L, Shen R, et al. Decreased peripheral mitochondrial DNA copy number is associated with the risk of heart failure and long-term outcomes. Medicine 2016;95(15):e3323.

48. Ellis G, Whitehead MA, Robinson D, et al. Comprehensive geriatric assessment for older adults admitted to hospital: meta-analysis of randomised controlled trials. BMJ 2011;343:d6553.

49. Martin FC, Brighton P. Frailty: different tools for different purposes? Age Ageing 2008;37(2):129–31.

50. Gielen E, Verschueren S, O'Neill T, et al. Musculoskeletal frailty: a geriatric syndrome at the core of fracture occurrence in older age. Calcif Tissue Int 2012; 91(3):161–77.

51. Karunananthan S, Wolfson C, Bergman H, et al. A multidisciplinary systematic literature review on frailty: overview of the methodology used by the Canadian initiative on frailty and aging. BMC Med Res Methodol 2009;9(1):1.

52. De Vries N, Staal J, Van Ravensberg C, et al. Outcome instruments to measure frailty: a systematic review. Ageing Res Rev 2011;10(1):104–14.

53. Dent E, Kowal P, Hoogendijk EO. Frailty measurement in research and clinical practice: a review. Eur J Intern Med 2016;31:3–10.

54. Rolfson DB, Majumdar SR, Tsuyuki RT, et al. Validity and reliability of the Edmonton Frail Scale. Age Ageing 2006;35(5):526–9.

55. Gobbens RJ, van Assen MA, Luijkx KG, et al. The Tilburg frailty indicator: psychometric properties. J Am Med Dir Assoc 2010;11(5):344–55.

56. Raîche M, Hébert R, Dubois MF. PRISMA-7: a case-finding tool to identify older adults with moderate to severe disabilities. Arch Gerontol Geriatr 2008;47(1): 9–18.

57. Steverink N, Slaets J, Schuurmans H, et al. Measuring frailty. Development and testing of the Groningen Frailty Indicator (GFI). Gerontologist 2001;41(1):236.

58. Habert R, Bravo G, Korner-Bitensky N, et al. Predictive validity of a postal questionnaire for screening community-dwelling elderly individuals at risk of functional decline. Age Ageing 1996;25(2):159–67.

59. Saliba D, Elliott M, Rubenstein LZ, et al. The vulnerable elders survey: a tool for identifying vulnerable older people in the community. J Am Geriatr Soc 2001; 49(12):1691–9.

60. Salvi F, Morichi V, Grilli A, et al. Screening for frailty in elderly emergency department patients by using the identification of seniors at risk (ISAR). J Nutr Health Aging 2012;16(4):313–8.

61. Sager MA, Rudberg MA, Jalaluddin M, et al. Hospital Admission Risk Profile (HARP): identifying older patients at risk for functional decline following acute medical illness and hospitalization. J Am Geriatr Soc 1996;44(3):251–7.

62. Guralnik JM, Simonsick EM, Ferrucci L, et al. A short physical performance battery assessing lower extremity function: association with self-reported disability and prediction of mortality and nursing home admission. J Gerontol 1994; 49(2):M85–94.

63. Morley JE, Malmstrom T, Miller D. A simple frailty questionnaire (FRAIL) predicts outcomes in middle aged African Americans. J Nutr Health Aging 2012;16(7): 601–8.
64. Vellas B, Balardy L, Gillette-Guyonnet S, et al. Looking for frailty in community-dwelling older persons: the Gérontopôle Frailty Screening Tool (GFST). J Nutr Health Aging 2013;17(7):629–31.
65. de Labra C, Guimaraes-Pinheiro C, Maseda A, et al. Effects of physical exercise interventions in frail older adults: a systematic review of randomized controlled trials. BMC Geriatr 2015;15(1):1.
66. Hopman P, de Bruin SR, Forjaz MJ, et al. Effectiveness of comprehensive care programs for patients with multiple chronic conditions or frailty: a systematic literature review. Health Policy 2016;120(7):818–32.
67. Jadczak AD, Makwana N, Luscombe-Marsh ND, et al. Effectiveness of exercise interventions on physical function in community-dwelling frail older people: an umbrella review protocol. JBI Database System Rev Implement Rep 2016; 14(9):93–102.
68. Wilson MG, Béland F, Julien D, et al. Interventions for preventing, delaying the onset, or decreasing the burden of frailty: an overview of systematic reviews. Syst Rev 2015;4:128.
69. Cadore EL, Rodríguez-Mañas L, Sinclair A, et al. Effects of different exercise interventions on risk of falls, gait ability, and balance in physically frail older adults: a systematic review. Rejuvenation Res 2013;16(2):105–14.
70. Theou O, Stathokostas L, Roland KP, et al. The effectiveness of exercise interventions for the management of frailty: a systematic review. J Aging Res 2011;2011: 569194.
71. Daniels R, van Rossum E, de Witte L, et al. Interventions to prevent disability in frail community-dwelling elderly: a systematic review. BMC Health Serv Res 2008;8:278.
72. Organization WH. Switzerland (Geniva): World Health Organization; Global recommendations on physical activity for health. 2010.
73. Devereux-Fitzgerald A, Powell R, Dewhurst A, et al. The acceptability of physical activity interventions to older adults: a systematic review and meta-synthesis. Soc Sci Med 2016;158:14–23.
74. Pate RR, Pratt M, Blair SN, et al. Physical activity and public health: a recommendation from the centers for disease control and prevention and the American College of Sports Medicine. JAMA 1995;273(5):402–7.
75. Walker S, Häkkinen K. Similar increases in strength after short-term resistance training due to different neuromuscular adaptations in young and older men. J Strength Cond Res 2014;28(11):3041–8.
76. Frimel TN, Sinacore DR, Villareal DT. Exercise attenuates the weight-loss-induced reduction in muscle mass in frail obese older adults. Med Sci Sports Exerc 2008; 40(7):1213.
77. Angulo J, El Assar M, Rodríguez-Mañas L. Frailty and sarcopenia as the basis for the phenotypic manifestation of chronic diseases in older adults. Mol Aspects Med 2016;50:1–32.
78. Nicholson C, Morrow EM, Hicks A, et al. Supportive care for older people with frailty in hospital: an integrative review. Int J Nurs Stud 2017;66:60–71.
79. Gill TM, Allore HG, Gahbauer EA, et al. Change in disability after hospitalization or restricted activity in older persons. JAMA 2010;304(17):1919–28.

Cognitive Issues
Decline, Delirium, Depression, Dementia

Melodee Harris, PhD, APRN, GNP-BC

KEYWORDS

- Decline • Delirium • Depression • Dementia

KEY POINTS

- Baseline cognitive status is important in the assessment of decline associated with delirium, depression, and dementia.
- Use screening tools that are valid for older persons.
- Early identification of symptoms and treatment of neurocognitive disorders prevent decline, disability, and mortality.
- Promote optimal independent functioning in older persons with neurocognitive disorders.

Cognitive decline in older persons can be pathologic or occur as a part of the normal aging process. Delirium, depression, and dementia are geriatric syndromes and neurocognitive disorders that are the result of cognitive decline associated with pathology.[1]

Cognition is the ability to acquire knowledge and mental awareness that allows interaction with the environment.[2] Age-related cognitive changes develop normally across the life span and are not pathologic.[3] In normal cognitive aging, memory is intact, but with slower recall.[3] There is also decline in visuoperceptual and visuospatial function.[3] Normal aging occurs with some loss of capacity for problem solving, known as fluid ability.[3] However, crystalized intelligence, such as verbal abilities, are more preserved.[3] Neuroimaging of normal aging may show patterns of diffuse, neurotic plaques that are sparsely distributed in the brain without any indication of dementia or other pathologic disorders.[4]

There are 2 categories of cognitive impairment: cognitive impairment no dementia (CIND) and mild cognitive impairment (MCI). CIND and MCI have a prevalence rates up to 39%.[5] Little is known about cognitive impairment because older persons tend to seek help when there is significant cognitive and functional decline that is more characteristic of dementia.

College of Nursing, University of Arkansas for Medical Sciences, 4301 West Markham Street, Slot #539, Little Rock, AR 72205, USA
E-mail address: harrismelodee@uams.edu

Nurs Clin N Am 52 (2017) 363–374
http://dx.doi.org/10.1016/j.cnur.2017.05.001
0029-6465/17/© 2017 Elsevier Inc. All rights reserved.

nursing.theclinics.com

All cognitive decline demands an explanation. The transition of normal age-related changes to pathology presents with an interruption in activities of daily living. Deficits in daily memory and executive function are the strongest predictors for the transition of normal age-related changes to cognitive impairment.[6]

This overview is a brief guide on cognitive decline and how to identify, manage, and treat associated neurocognitive disorders including delirium, depression, and dementia.

DELIRIUM
Definition

Delirium is a neurocognitive disorder[1] and a geriatric syndrome.[7] Delirium has an atypical presentation.[8] Delirium is characterized by inattention with a sudden onset of cognitive decline and fluctuating course alternating with lucidness.[8,9]

Delirium Subtypes

Delirium has 3 basic presentations: hyperactive, hypoactive, and mixed subtypes. Health care providers tend to recognize the hyperactive subtype of delirium because of its sudden onset and severe agitation. Somnolence is the typical presentation of the hypoactive subtype and is often underdiagnosed. The mixed subtype of delirium fluctuates between severe agitation and somnolence. Mixed delirium also is overlooked by clinicians.[9]

Prognosis

Delirium occurs in 1 in 5 hospitalized older persons, with the highest prevalence in neurology units and the lowest prevalence on rehabilitation units.[10]

There is an 18% prevalence rate and a 56% rate of incidence of delirium in persons with dementia.[8] There is a 32% prevalence rate of delirium superimposed on dementia in the hospital.[11]

The consequences of delirium include prolonged hospitalization, functional decline, and mortality.

Risk Factors

Hospitalization places older persons at risk for delirium. Iatrogenic causes of delirium in the intensive care unit (ICU) include mechanical ventilation, sedating medications, and immobilization.[12]

Geriatric Assessment

Important Overall Consideration: Assess Baseline Cognitive Status in Older Persons.

Screening

There are multiple reliable and valid tools to screen older persons for delirium. The Confusion Assessment Method (CAM) has a 94% to 100% sensitivity and an 89% to 95% specificity.[13,14] The CAM-ICU has a sensitivity of 93% to 100% and a specificity of 93% to 100%.[15] Other screening tools are the Delirium Symptom Interview, Nursing Delirium Screening and the Intensive Care Delirium Screening Check List.[16]

Assess, Treat, and Manage Underlying, Causes

- Consider cardiovascular causes such as congestive heart failure of myocardial infarction[7–9]
- Consider neurologic causes such as CVA stroke[8]

- Minimize pain[7]
- Correct dehydration[7–9]
- Correct electrolyte imbalance[7–9]
- Manage hypo/hyperglycemia[8]
- Minimize sensory Impairment[7,9]
- Treat infections[7,9]
- Eliminate polypharmacy[7,8]
- Eliminate environmental causes[7,8]
- Discontinue catheters as soon as possible[7]

Pharmacology

There is insufficient evidence for or against using antipsychotic medications in the treatment of delirium. Antipsychotic medications are used when there are safety concerns or to relieve severe psychosis.[16] However, antipsychotic medications should be used with caution in older persons with dementia. Benzodiazepines cause confusion and should not be used as a first-line treatment for delirium.[16] Once thought to be effective, cholinesterase inhibitors should not be newly prescribed to manage delirium.[16]

Disease Complications

Complications of delirium include physical, mental, and cognitive decline; institutionalization; and death in older persons.[8] Persistent delirium can last for months and years. The consequences of undiagnosed and untreated delirium results in permanent neuronal damage and dementia.[17] The national cost of direct care for delirium over 1 year is estimated from $143 billion to $152 billion.[18] The annual costs for facility, provider, and pharmacy were $9565 an older person with delirium superimposed on dementia and $7566 in dementia alone.[19] Outcomes are more severe when delirium is superimposed on dementia.[11] Older persons with dementia experience approximately 1 to 8 days in delirium, lower scores on the Katz Index of Independence in Activities of Daily Living, and higher scores on the Geriatric Depression Scale.[11]

Delirium superimposed on dementia is often unrecognized and undiagnosed.[11] Delirium screening is especially important in persons with dementia. Early recognition of delirium not only decreases hospital cost, but more importantly, saves lives.[20]

Evidence

One evidence-based practice to reduce delirium is the *A*wakening and *B*reathing *C*oordination, *D*elirium monitoring/management, and *E*arly exercise/mobility (ABCDE Bundle).[12] The ABCDE Bundle is an effective tool for monitoring and reducing patient respiratory status during mechanical ventilation and delirium, as well as early mobilization to reduce hospital stays.[12]

Controversies

Delirium has not been studied in specific populations. Persons with dementia have been excluded from research studies. Results for cognitive impairment that show up on screening for delirium may be confounded by dementia. In addition, it is difficult to identify if dementia is superimposed on delirium and the severity of delirium. Biomarker studies on delirium, such as inflammatory markers, are also needed.[21,22]

Delirium Rooms are one strategy that requires further research in older persons. Delirium Rooms are used to promote awareness of delirium. Strategies include

24-hour nursing monitoring, protocols for early mobility, enhanced lighting, and decreased sensory stimulation.[23]

Severe agitation is a consequence of delirium, and older persons who are at risk for self-harm may require antipsychotic medications. Because of adverse side effects, antipsychotic medications should be used with caution in older persons. If administered at all, prescriptions need to be at the lowest possible dose for the maximum effect.[24]

DEPRESSION
Definition

Depression is a mood disorder that also can cause cognitive decline. However, depression is not the result of normal aging. There are no specific *Diagnostic and Statistical Manual of Mental Disorders, 5th Edition* (DSM-5)[1] criteria for depression in older persons.

Diagnostic and Statistical Manual of Mental Disorders, 5th Edition Criteria for Depression

Depressed mood or loss of interest in pleasure is included in 5 or more of the symptoms listed as follows. The symptoms are during the same 2-week interval and associated with deterioration in baseline function.

1. Depressed mood most of the day or almost every day (sadness, emptiness, hopelessness) or
2. Loss of interest or pleasure every day or nearly every day in all or almost all activities.
3. Unintended weight loss or weight gain (5% of body weight in a month).
4. Psychomotor agitation or retardation almost every day.
5. Fatigue or loss of energy every day.
6. Feelings of worthlessness, or excessive or inappropriate guilt almost every day.
7. Decreased ability to think, concentrate, or make a decision almost every day.
8. Recurrent thoughts of death or suicidal ideation. May be without a specific plan or attempt.

These symptoms are clinically distressing or cause impairment in social, occupational, or other areas of functioning. The symptoms must not be explained by another physical or mental illness.

Atypical Presentations

Older persons may present with symptoms of depression. Older persons may demonstrate apathy, fatigue, somatic complaints, sleep disturbances, anger out of proportion to incident, and other atypical presentations rather than tearfulness or sadness.[25]

Prognosis

Depression is one of the most common geriatric mental health conditions. Compared with the general adult population, the prevalence of depression is lower in older adults.[26] The prevalence of major depressive disorder doubles in older women and in persons 70 to 85 years old. There are higher rates of depression in acute care and nursing home settings than in the community. Less severe symptoms of depression are higher than major depressive disorder in older persons. Older adults with less severe symptoms of depression may continue to remain depressed after 1 year[27–29] (Table 1).

Table 1 Prevalence of depression in older persons			
Major Depressive Disorder		**Other Depressive Symptoms/Disorders[a]**	
Older Adults[28,29]	1%–4%	Community[28]	8%–16%
White[27]	3.5%	White[27]	3.8%
African American[27]	3.4%	African American[27]	3.6%
Hispanic Latino[27]	6.1%	Hispanic Latino[27]	6.9%
Hospital[26]	10%–12%	Hospital[26]	8%–>40%
Nursing home[26]	12%–20%	Nursing home[28,29]	17%–35%

[a] Subclinical, subsyndromal, minor depression or depressive disorders.
Data from Refs.[26–29]

Risk Factors

Chronic illnesses, including diabetes, cardiovascular disease, osteoarthritis, and neurologic conditions, are risk factors for depression.[30,31] Sensory deficits, especially in older persons who are hard of hearing, are risk factors for depression. Loneliness and functional decline also place older persons at risk.[32]

Screening

Valid tools for older persons should be used to screen for depression (**Table 2**).

Table 2 Screening tools for depression		
PHQ-9	9 questions	DSM and symptoms of depression
PHQ-2	2 questions	1. Sadness 2. Anhedonia
Geriatric Depression Scale	15 items or Short Form	Does not screen for suicidal ideation
Cornell Scale for Depression in Dementia	19 items	Observational: caregiver and clinician

Abbreviations: DSM, Diagnostic and Statistical Manual of Mental Disorders; PHQ, Patient Health Questionnaire.
Data from Byrd EH, Vito NA. Nursing assessment and treatment of depressive disorders of late life. In: Melillo KD, Houde SC, editors. Geropsychiatric and mental health nursing. 2nd edition. Sudbury (MA): Jones & Bartlett Learning, LLC; 2011. p. 147–74.

Complications

The poor outcomes associated with depression include worsening physical conditions, functional decline, disability, institutionalization, and decreased quality of life. The worst outcome is suicide. Compared with other populations, adults 75 years and older have the highest rate of suicide.[33]

Treatment and Management

For maximum results, older persons with major depressive disorder should be treated with pharmacologic therapy in conjunction with cognitive therapies.[34] Nonpharmacological treatments, such as exercise, social activities, journaling, art therapy, and complementary and alternative therapies, can be included in treatment for depression.[35,36] Spiritual assessment is an overlooked approach in the plan of care for depression. Like younger adults, pharmacologic therapy may be implemented. The dose of an antidepressant for an older person should be prescribed at one-third to one-half that of a healthy adult.[37] Close monitoring is required, as it may take 4 weeks to identify if an antidepressant will be effective and 12 weeks to for remission of symptoms in an older person[26] (Table 3).

Table 3 Antidepressants		
Selective serotonin reuptake inhibitors (SSRI)	Citalopram Escitalopram Sertraline	Citalopram QT prolongation >20 mg Hyponatremia; serotonin syndrome
Selective serotonergic and noradrenergic reuptake inhibitors (SSRI/SNRI)	Duloxetine Venlafaxine	Dose adjustments; renal insufficiency Hypertension; Taper dosage
Tricyclic antidepressant (TCA)	Nortriptyline	Avoid in older persons
Noradrenergic and specific serotonergic antidepressants (NaSSA)	Mirtazapine	Benefits to older persons are decreased symptoms of depression, increased appetite, and sleep

Modified from Resnick B. Depression and mood disorders. Geriatric Nursing Review Syllabus. 2016. p. 322–9; with permission.

Controversies

Collaborative Care Models are used in the successful treatment of depression in older persons. Comparative effectiveness research shows that the integration of behavioral health into primary care improves geriatric mental health care including minority groups[38] The US Preventive Task Force recommends routine screenings and treatment for depression.[39] Nevertheless, these recommendations are not routinely implemented. Mental health disparities continue for older persons. More research is needed on social determinants and mental health disparities in older persons.[32]

DEMENTIA

Dementia is the most well-known neurocognitive disorder that is associated with cognitive decline in older persons. Cognitive function should be evaluated at baseline, admission, and ongoing.[40] Memory, executive functioning, and visual spatial ability is an important element in the promotion of functional independence.[40]

Definition

Dementia is a neurocognitive disorder[1] and geriatric syndrome of cognitive decline.[41] Dementia includes memory loss that interferes with daily functioning. The DSM-5[1] distinguishes among mild cognitive impairment, mild neurocognitive disorder, and major neurocognitive disorder.[42]

The DSM-5 identifies cognitive domains in relationship to cognitive impairment rather than the previous terminology: amnesia aphasia, apraxia, and agnosia. Cognitive domains include complex attention, executive function, learning and memory, language, and perceptual motor and social cognition.[1,2]

Mild neurocognitive disorder is a decrease in cognitive function that is beyond normal aging. Mild neurocognitive disorder may or may not transition to dementia.[42] Major neurocognitive disorder refers to all syndromes of dementia.[42,43]

Prognosis

It is estimated that 5.4 million Americans have a diagnosis of Alzheimer dementia. One (11%) in 9 persons age 65 and older have Alzheimer dementia (Table 4).[44]

Table 4
Overview of dementia syndromes

Dementia Subtype	Epidemiology	Pathology	Trajectory
Alzheimer dementia	60%–80%	Genetic-Apolipoprotein E (APOE-e4) Beta-amyloid plaque	Slow, gradual progression
Vascular dementia	10% 50% older persons	Blood vessel damage Infarcts	Stair-step progression
Dementia with Lewy body	—	Alpha-synuclein	Aggressive progression
Parkinson dementia	1/10th of Alzheimer disease	Lewy body Beta-amyloid clumps Tau tangles	Gradual progression
Frontotemporal lobar degeneration (FLD)	10% 60% 45–60 y old	Tau or transactive response DNA binding protein	Younger onset
Normal-pressure hydrocephalus	<5%	Build up cerebrospinal fluid	Memory loss with incontinence and gait instability

Data from Alzheimer's Association. 2016 Alzheimer's facts and figures. Washington, DC: Author; 2016 12(4), **Table 2** Causes of Dementia and Associated Characteristics p. 6–7 and Resnick B. Dementia. Geriatric nursing review syllabus. 5th edition. New York: American Geriatrics Society; 2016. p. 280–91.

Risk Factors, Assessment, Screening

Age itself is a risk factor for dementia. However, the transition from MCI to dementia is heralded by depression, executive dysfunction, and neuropsychiatric symptoms. A poor response to treatment for depression in older persons with MCI is a risk factor for dementia. Executive dysfunction is the inability to make decisions and predicts the severity of neuropsychiatric symptoms. Examples of neuropsychiatric symptoms include apathy, mood disorders, irritability, agitation, and psychosis. Poor diet is also recognized as a risk factor for dementia[42] (**Table 5**).

Table 5
Geriatric assessment and screening tools

Assessment Categories	Screening Tools
Cognition	Clock Drawing Minicog
Function	Katz Index of Independence in Activities of Daily Living Lawton-Brody Independent Activities of Daily Living
Behavioral assessment	Geriatric Depression Scale
Physical assessment	History and physical Family, social, environmental Laboratory testing: complete blood count, basic metabolic panel, liver panel, thyroid panel, B12, folate, rapid plasma reagin testing Imaging: noncontrast computed tomography and MRI
Environmental	Home safety and fall risk
Caregiver assessment	Caregiver stress

Adapted from Fletcher K. Dementia: a neurocognitive disorder. In: Boltz M, Capezuti E, Fulmer T, et al, editors. Evidence based geriatric nursing protocols for best practice. New York: Spring Publishing Company, LLC; 2016. p. 443–67.

Complications

Functional decline may predict poor outcomes in persons with dementia and end-stage chronic illness. Dementia predicates loss of independence, institutionalization, morbidity, mortality, and decreased quality of life.

Treatment Options: Brief Overview

Key concept: individualize

Effective interventions are multimodal, but should be individualized, and person-centered and family-centered. Safety is a priority. The plan of care should be interprofessional with the older person as the central team member. Assess, evaluate, treat, manage, and monitor all treatment options.[45,46]

Older persons with major neurocognitive disorder have a higher rate of multiple chronic illnesses. In fact, a diagnosis of diabetes, hypertension, obesity, or cardiovascular disease may be the underlying cause of dementia.[46] The close management of chronic illnesses may prevent or slow the disease process.

There are only 4 medications that are approved by the Food and Drug Administration for major neurocognitive disorders. Drug classes are cholinesterase inhibitors and N-methyl-D-aspartate (NMDA) receptor antagonists. Cholinesterase inhibitors are cognitive-enhancing medications, such as donepezil, rivastigmine, and galantamine. Cholinesterase inhibitors are given to place the disease process in remission and optimize function in activities of daily living for as long as possible. Memantine is an NMDA receptor antagonist that can be used in conjunction with cholinesterase inhibitors. Memantine is usually given for middle-stage dementia.[46–48]

A holistic nonpharmacological approach should be implemented as a first-line intervention for major neurocognitive disorders. The environment is most significant and should be restraint free with scheduled routines and anticipation of needs. Complementary and alternative therapies, such as aromatherapy, music, and art therapy, have few side effects and may be beneficial in reducing behavioral and psychological symptoms of dementia.[46]

Behavioral interventions designed to manage depression, anxiety, and mental illness should be considered to prevent further cognitive and functional decline and improve quality of life.

Social interventions include case management for resources that allow optimal independence, such as public transportation or meal services. Legal consultation with a representative who specializes in geriatric care can help patients and families to maximize assets and advise on advance directives.[46]

Finally, caregivers also require therapeutic interventions. Education and respite care should be encouraged. Support groups often provide socialization and unique caregiver resources.

Evidence

The goals for treatment in older persons with dementia include safety, optimal function, and quality of life. Some evidence for nonpharmacological treatment is based on inconsistent or limited quality person-oriented evidence from smaller cohort studies or randomized controlled trials.[26] Nonpharmacological treatments should be implemented, such as environmental modification, family education and support. Pharmacologic treatments, such as cholinesterase inhibitors, should be followed closely for benefit and adverse side effects.[46] Antipsychotic medications are not recommended for older persons with dementia and behavioral symptoms.[49]

Controversies

Research is needed on the transition from mild neurocognitive disorder to dementia, as most research is based on MCI. Neuropsychiatric symptoms are common in mild neurocognitive disorder; however, there is little research on treatment for neuropsychiatric symptoms in older persons with mild neurocognitive disorder.[42] Additionally, more research is needed on genetics, biomarkers, and nonpharmacologic interventions in the treatment of dementia.

SUMMARY

In 2010, there were 40.3 million older persons.[50] By 2030, there will be 74 million persons older than 65.[51] In 2050, there will be 88 million older persons and 98 million by 2060.[51] The incidence rates of cognitive decline associated with neurocognitive disorders will continue to grow. Primary care providers are challenged to identify, assess, manage, treat, and prevent cognitive decline associated with delirium, depression, and dementia. The expert management of cognitive decline associated with neurocognitive disorders is an important skillset that will make a difference and improve quality of life for the geriatric population.

REFERENCES

1. American Psychiatric Association. Diagnostic and statistical manual of mental disorders. 5th edition. Arlington (VA): American Psychiatric Association; 2013.
2. Kimchi EZ, Lyketsos CG. Dementia and mild neurocognitive disorders. In: Blazer DG, Steffens DC, editors. The American Psychiatric Publishing textbook of geriatric psychiatry. Washington, DC: American Psychiatric Publishing; 2015. p. 240–322.
3. Welsh-Bohmer KA, Attix DK. Neuropsychological assessment of late-life cognitive disorders. In: Steffens DC, Blazer DG, Thakur ME, editors. Psychiatric Publishing textbook of geriatric psychiatry. Washington, DC: American Psychiatric Publishing; 2015. p. 178–210.
4. Taylor WD, Moore SD, Chin SS. Neuroanatomy, neurophysiology, and neuropathology of aging. In: Blazer DG, Steffens DC, editors. The American Psychiatric Publishing textbook of geriatric psychiatry. Washington, DC: American Psychiatric Publishing; 2009. p. 63–94.
5. Hybels CF, Moore SD, Chin SS. Neuropsycholoigal assessment of late-life cognitive disorders. In: Blazer DG, Steffens DC, editors. The American Psychiatric Publishing textbook of geriatric psychiatry. Washington, DC: American Psychiatric Publishing; 2015. p. 178–210.
6. Farias ST, Lau K, Harvey D, et al. Early functional limitations in cognitively normal older adults predict diagnostic conversion to mild cognitive impairment. J Am Geriatr Soc 2017;1–7. http://dx.doi.org/10.1111/jgs.14835.
7. Tullmann DF, Blevins C, Fletcher K. Delirium: prevention, early recognition, and treatment. In: Boltz M, Capezuti E, Fulmer T, et al, editors. Evidence-based geriatric nursing protocols for best practice. 5th edition. New York: Springer Publishing; 2016. p. 408–87.
8. Inouye SK, Westendorp R, Saczynski J. Delirium in elderly people. Lancet 2014; 383(9920):911–22.
9. Saczynski JS, Inouye SK. Delirium. In: Steffens DC, Blazer DG, Thakur ME, editors. Psychiatric Publishing textbook of geriatric psychiatry. Washington, DC: American Psychiatric Publishing; 2015. p. 212–39.

10. Bellelli G, Morandi A, Di Santo SG, et al. "Delirium Day": a nationwide point prevalence study of delirium in older hospitalized patients using an easy standardized diagnostic tool. BMC Med 2016;14:106.
11. Fick DM, Steis MR, Waller JL, et al. Delirium superimposed on dementia is associated with prolonged length of stay and poor outcomes in hospitalized older adults. J Hosp Med 2013;8(9):500–5.
12. Balas MC, Vasilevskis EE, Olsen KM, et al. Effectiveness and safety of the awakening and breathing coordination, delirium monitoring/management and early exercise/mobility (ABCDE) bundle. Crit Care Med 2014;42(5):1024–36.
13. Wei LA, Fearing MA, Eliezer J, et al. The confusion assessment method (CAM): a systematic review of current usage. J Am Geriatr Soc 2008;56(5):823–30.
14. Waszynski C. The Confusion Assessment Method (CAM). Try This 2012, 13. Available at: https://consultgeri.org/try-this/general-assessment/issue-13.pdf. Accessed June 14, 2017.
15. Tate JA, Happ MG. The Confusion Assessment Method ICU (CAM-ICU). Try This. 2012, 25. Available at: https://consultgeri.org/try-this/general-assessment/issue-25.pdf. Accessed June 14, 2017.
16. Inouye SK, Robinson T, Blaum C, et al. Postoperative delirium in older adults: best practice statement from the American Geriatrics Society. J Am Coll Surg 2015; 220(2):136–48.e1.
17. Fong TG, Davis D, Growdon ME, et al. The interface of delirium and dementia in older persons. Lancet Neurol 2015;14(8):823–32.
18. Leslie DL, Inouye SK. The importance of delirium: economic and societal costs. J Am Geriatr Soc 2011;59(Suppl 2):S241–3.
19. Fick D, Kolanowski A, Waller JL, et al. Delirium superimposed on dementia in a community-dwelling managed care population: a 3-year retrospective study of occurrence, costs, and utilization. J Gerontol 2005;60A(6):748–53.
20. Richards R. Delirium: the 21st century health care challenge for bedside clinicians. J Nurs Educ Pract 2015;6(6):8–16.
21. Davis DH, Kreisel SH, Muniz Terrera G, et al. The epidemiology of delirium: challenges and opportunities for population studies. Am J Geriatr Psychiatry 2013;21: 1173–89.
22. Kahn BA, Zawahiri M, Campbell NL, et al. Biomarkers for delirium–a review. J Am Geriatr Soc 2011;59(0 2):S256–81.
23. Flaherty JH, Steele DK, Chibnall JT, et al. An ACE unit with a delirium room may improve function and equalize length of stay among older delirious medical inpatients. J Gerontol A Biol Sci Med Sci 2010;65A(12):1387–92.
24. Inouye SK, Marcantonio ER, Metzger ED. Doing damage in delirium: the hazards of antipsychotic treatment in elderly persons. Lancet Psychiatry 2013;1(4):312–5.
25. Wiese BS. Geriatric depression: the use of antidepressants in the elderly. BCMJ 2011;53(7):341–7.
26. Resnick B. Depression and mood disorders. Geriatric nursing review syllabus. New York: American Geriatrics Society; 2016. p. 322–9.
27. Institute of Medicine. The mental health and substance use work-force for older adults: in whose hands? Washington, DC: National Academies Press; 2012.
28. Blazer DG. Depression in late life: review and commentary. J Gerontol A Biol Sci Med Sci 2003;58(3):249–65.
29. Alexopoulos GS. Depression in the elderly. Lancet 2005;365:1961–70.
30. Fiske A, Wetherell JL, Gatz M. Depression in older adults. Ann Rev Clin Psychol 2009;5:363–89.

31. Karp JF, Dew MA, Wahed AS, et al. Challenges and solutions for depression prevention research: methodology for a depression prevention trial for older adults with knee arthritis and emotional distress. Am J Geriatr Psychiatry 2016;24(6): 433–43.

32. Tanner EK, Martinez IL, Harris M. Examining functional and social determinants of depression in community-dwelling older adults: implications for practice. Geriatr Nurs 2014;35:236–40.

33. Curtin SC, Warner M, Hedegaard H. Increase in suicide in the United States, 1999-2015. NCHS Data Brief 2016;241:1–7. Available at: https://www.cdc.gov/nchs/data/databriefs/db241.pdf.

34. Siu AL, the US Preventive Services Task Force (USPSTF). Screening for depression in adults: US Preventive Task Force recommendation statement. JAMA 2016; 315(4):380–7.

35. Simmons M, Peraza-Smith GB, Harris M, et al. Application of resources for non-pharmacological interventions to improve dementia care in nursing homes. Geriatr Nurs 2015;36(3):242–4.

36. Resnick B. Research review: exercise interventions for treatment of depression. Geriatr Nurs 2005;26(3):196.

37. Khouzam HR. Depression in the elderly: how to treat. Consultant 360 2012;52:4.

38. Community Preventive Services Task Force. Improving mental health and addressing mental illness: collaborative care for the management of depressive disorders. 2014. Available at: https://www.thecommunityguide.org/sites/default/files/assets/Mental-Health-Collaborative-Care.pdf. Accessed June 14, 2017.

39. Final Recommendation Statement. Depression in adults: screening. U.S. Preventive Services Task Force; 2016. Available at: https://www.uspreventiveservicestaskforce.org/Page/Document/RecommendationStatementFinal/depression-in-adults-screening1.

40. Boltz M, Resnick B, Galik E. Preventing functional decline in the acute care setting. In: Boltz M, Capezuti E, Fulmer T, et al, editors. Evidence based geriatric nursing protocols for best practice. New York: Spring Publishing Company, LLC; 2016. p. 368–91.

41. Fletcher K. Dementia: a neurocognitive disorder. In: Boltz M, Capezuti E, Fulmer T, et al, editors. Evidence based geriatric nursing protocols for best practice. New York: Spring Publishing Company, LLC; 2016. p. 443–67.

42. Sachs-Ericsson N, Blazer DG. The new DSM-5 diagnosis of mild neurocognitive disorder and its relation to research in mild cognitive impairment. Aging Ment Health 2016;19(12):2–12. Available at: http://dx.doi.org/10.1080/13607863.2014.920303.

43. Alzheimer's Association. 2016 Alzheimer's facts and figures. Washington, DC: Author; 2016.

44. Alzheimer's Association. 2016 Alzheimer's disease facts and figures. Alzheimers Dement 2016;12(4):1–80.

45. Lyketsos CG. The evaluation and formulation of dementia. In: Rabins PV, Lyketsos CG, Steele CD, editors. Practical dementia care. 3rd edition. New York: Oxford University Press; 2016. p. 61–89.

46. Plank LM. Dementia. In: Kennedy-Malone L, Fletcher KR, Plank LM, editors. Advanced practice nursing in the care of older adults. Philadelphia: FA Davis; 2013. p. 562–72.

47. Alzheimer's disease medication fact sheet. Bethesda (MD): NIH Publication; 2016. No 16-AG-3431.

48. Birks JS. Cholinesterase inhibitors for Alzheimer's disease. Cochrane Database Syst Rev 2006;(1):CD005593.
49. Reus VI, Fochtmann LJ, Eyler AE, et al. The American Psychiatric Association practice guideline on the use of antipsychotics to treat agitation or psychosis in patients with dementia. Am J Psychiatry 2016;173:543–6.
50. Vincent GK, Velkoff VA. The next four decades: the older population in the United States: 2010 to 2050. Current population reports. Washington, DC: U.S. Census Bureau; 2010. p. 25–1138.
51. Colby SL, Ortman JM. Projections of the size and composition of the U.S. population: 2014 to 2060. Current population reports. Washington, DC: U.S. Census Bureau; 2014. p. 25–1143.

Pain Assessment in Older Adults

Ann L. Horgas, RN, PhD, FGSA

KEYWORDS

- Pain • Pain management • Older adults • Barriers • Cognitive impairment

KEY POINTS

- Pain is a common symptom experienced by older adults.
- Pain is a complex phenomenon with multiple causes and consequences.
- Pain assessment is a critical step in developing a pain management plan.
- Assessment of pain should reply on self-report and other pain indicators.

INTRODUCTION

Pain is a common experience for many older adults. Elderly adults, particularly those ages 85 and older, are the fastest growing segment of the US population. Longer life, however, does not necessarily mean disease-free or symptom-free years. Aging increases the risk of pain due to the high rate of chronic and acute conditions; 45% of Medicare beneficiaries have at least 4 chronic conditions.[1] In 2010, 13.6 million adults older than 65 were discharged from an acute care hospital and 298.4 million visited an ambulatory care clinic at least once.[2] In the same year, more than 19 million surgeries were performed on older adults, including 5.2 million musculoskeletal surgeries (including knee and hip replacements).[2] Thus, pain is not only common, but also a somewhat complex phenomenon among older adults.

BACKGROUND

Before the mid-1990s, very little attention was paid to geriatric pain in the clinical or empirical literature. Since then, significant efforts have been undertaken to address and improve the assessment and management of pain in older adults. In 2001, the Joint Commission on Accreditation of Healthcare Organizations declared pain the "fifth vital sign," and mandated pain assessment and management be evaluated as part of the hospital accreditation process.[3] This mandate exposed some of the challenges associated with assessing and managing pain in older adults, particularly

Department of Biobehavioral Nursing Science, College of Nursing, University of Florida, PO Box 100197-HSC, Gainesville, FL 32610, USA
E-mail address: ahorgas@ufl.edu

Nurs Clin N Am 52 (2017) 375–385
http://dx.doi.org/10.1016/j.cnur.2017.04.006
0029-6465/17/© 2017 Elsevier Inc. All rights reserved.

among those with cognitive impairment who could not verbally express pain. This led to a proliferation of tools to assess pain in this population.[4,5] In addition, several clinical guidelines were established by such leading professional organizations as the American Geriatrics Society,[6,7] American Pain Society,[8] British Geriatric Society,[9] and the American Society for Pain Management Nursing.[10] In 2011, the Institute of Medicine published a report, *Relieving Pain in America: A Blueprint for Transforming Prevention, Care, Education, and Research*, that declared chronic pain in the United States as a public health problem due to the human and economic costs and the challenges of pain management.[11] The report provided recommendations for transforming the way pain is understood, assessed, treated, and prevented. In this report, older adults are considered at high risk for inadequate pain management. More recently, the Gerontological Society of America established policy recommendations to improving pain care.[12] These initiatives have heightened awareness of the problem of pain in older adults, yet there is compelling evidence that pain remains poorly assessed and managed.[13,14]

EPIDEMIOLOGY OF PAIN

The high prevalence of pain among older adults is well documented.[11,15] In a nationwide US survey, approximately 50% of older adults reported experiencing bothersome pain in the preceding month.[16] Estimates are higher in older adults with cognitive impairment and multiple comorbidities, such as those residing in long-term care facilities. In this setting, it is estimated that as many as 83% to 93% experience pain on a regular basis.[17] These prevalence estimates, however, provide a unidimensional picture of pain. Given the multimorbidity referenced previously, older adults commonly experience multiple causes and types of pain.[16]

A common question is whether the prevalence of pain increases with age. It is often assumed that old age is associated with pain. Certainly, there is an increased prevalence of conditions commonly associated with pain, such as osteoarthritis, in older adults. However, the evidence that they actually cause pain is equivocal. In the empirical literature, 4 relationship patterns have been identified.[17] These patterns can be characterized as follows: (1) linear increase (pain increases with age), (2) inverse relationship (pain increases until middle age [50–65 years] or old age [75–85 years] and then decreases), (3) linear decrease (pain diminishes with advancing age), or (4) no age differences.[17] The patterns vary across pain conditions.[17,18] Musculoskeletal pain (including back pain) appears to peak at midlife or old age and then decline in the oldest-old (older than 85 years) in some studies, but continues to increase with age in other studies. Headaches (eg, migraines and severe headaches), myocardial infarction–related pain, and cancer-related pain all appear to decrease with advancing age.[19] It is difficult to draw firm conclusions from these data because the studies differ in terms of the methodology used and the specificity with which they define the type of pain studied.[19] In addition, there are wide differences among older adults in their medical history and presentation and in the psychosocial factors that can influence the experience of pain. Thus, clinicians should rely on their diagnostic and clinical judgment when evaluating pain, and not be unduly biased by expectations of the pain experience among older adults.

CAUSES AND CONSEQUENCES OF PAIN IN OLDER ADULTS

Fig. 1 provides a conceptual framework for understanding some of the factors that contribute to pain in older adults, as well as the consequences of unrelieved pain. In addition, it highlights the relationship between acute and persistent pain. Each of

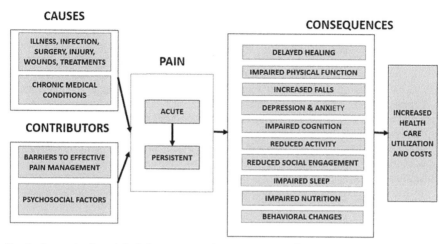

Fig. 1. Conceptual model of the causes and consequences of pain in older adults.

these constructs is discussed in the following sections, starting with the central construct of pain.

Definitions of Pain

The International Association of the Study of Pain (IASP) defines pain as "an unpleasant sensory and emotional experience associated with actual or potential tissue damage, or described in terms of such damage."[20] Pain is further defined as a complex, multidimensional, subjective experience with recognized sensory, cognitive, and emotional dimensions.[7,21] McCaffery[5,22] provides another classic definition of pain: "Pain is whatever the experiencing person says it is, existing whenever he says it does." These definitions highlight the highly subjective and multidimensional nature of pain, and the need for clinicians to rely on patient self-report to assess pain.

There are different types and characteristics of pain, prompting much scientific and clinical work to define taxonomies of pain. The IASP has taken the lead on this work (see IASP Taxonomy http://www.iasp-pain.org/Taxonomy). The most common distinctions define pain as acute or persistent (sometime referred to as chronic pain) and neuropathic or nociceptive. Distinctions are also made between cancer (malignant) and noncancer pain. The reader is encouraged to explore the full array of definitions and subcategories of pain on the IASP Web site. The Geriatric Pain Web site, hosted by Sigma Theta Tau International, also provides a useful and succinct summary of key terms and definitions (www.geriatricpain.org).

Causes and Types of Pain

Acute pain is typically associated with surgery, fractures, acute illness, or trauma.[23] Persistent pain (often referred to as chronic pain) is pain that persists past the usual healing time, typically defined as 3 months. The term persistent pain has been widely adopted in the literature because it is thought to reflect a more accurate, but more positive, representation of the nature of pain that requires long-term adaptation and management and is often not curable. *Persistent pain* is most frequently associated with common chronic diseases among older adults, such as cardiovascular disease, diabetes mellitus, degenerative joint disease, osteoporosis, cancer, and peripheral neuropathies.[24] *Nociceptive pain* is caused by actual or threatened damage to organs, skin, muscle, and bones (eg, non–nervous system tissue); pain results from the activation of nociceptors that process painful stimuli. Osteoarthritic back/neck pain is one of the most common types of nociceptive pain in older adults.[18] In contrast, *neuropathic pain* is caused by damage or disease directly affecting the somatosensory nervous system. There are 2 subtypes of neuropathic pain: central and peripheral. *Central neuropathic pain* is caused by disease or damage to the central somatosensory nervous system by conditions such as Parkinson disease, poststroke myelopathies, spinal cord injuries, spinal stenosis, multiple sclerosis, and fibromyalgia. *Peripheral neuropathic pain* is caused by conditions such as postherpetic neuralgia, metabolic disorders (eg, diabetic neuropathy, alcohol), nerve compression or entrapment, phantom limb pain, and trigeminal neuralgia.[25] Neuropathic pain is often associated with abnormal sensations (dysesthesia) or pain from normally nonpainful stimuli (allodynia), may be continuous and/or episodic, and is often characterized by tingling or stabbing sensations.

Older adults are at risk for experiencing multiple types of pain. When treating acute pain, health care providers should recognize the possibility that older adults also may be experiencing underlying persistent pain. These overlapping pain conditions may influence recovery and rehabilitation, particularly if pain impairs mobility that is vital to healing. It is also important to note the growing evidence that unrelieved acute pain may cause persistent pain. The strongest evidence for this relationship relates to the development of persistent postsurgical pain.[26] Severe acute pain after surgery has been shown to be a significant predictor for the development of persistent pain in adults who underwent lower extremity amputation, breast surgery, thoracotomy, inguinal hernia repair, coronary artery bypass surgery, and cholecystectomy,[27] all of which are common surgical procedures among older adults. These findings highlight the importance of effectively managing pain.

Other Factors that Contribute to Pain

Fig. 1 also highlights other factors that contribute to the experience of pain among older adults: barriers to effective pain management and psychosocial factors. Barriers to effective pain assessment and treatment fall into 3 domains: individual-based, provider-based, and system-based factors. *Individual-based factors* that may impair pain management include the following: (1) belief that pain is a normal part of aging, (2) concern of being labeled a hypochondriac or complainer, (3) fear of the meaning of pain in relation to disease progression or prognosis, (4) fear of opioid addiction and analgesics, (5) worry about health care costs, and (6) a belief that pain is not important to health care providers.[7] Cognitive impairment is also an important barrier because dementia reduces older adults' ability to remember and report pain.[13,28] *Provider-based factors* refer to knowledge deficits among nurses (and other health care providers) in effective pain management. Because there is no objective measure of pain, providers must rely on patients' self-report to assess pain. The evidence indicates that health care providers, in general, have a tendency to doubt or underestimate patients' reports of pain.[5] Among cognitively impaired older adults, several studies have documented that impaired individuals were prescribed and administered significantly less analgesic medication than were cognitively intact older adults.[29,30] This finding may reflect providers' difficulty detecting pain in persons who cannot verbally express its presence and lack of knowledge of pain management in this population. *System-based factors* refer to policies and regulations about prescription practices and prescriptive authority. Providers face strict regulations as to how opioids can be prescribed and who can prescribe them. In 2016, Florida became the final state to achieve controlled substance prescriptive authority for nurse practitioners. At the national level, the US federal government recently issued new regulations on prescribing in an effort to combat the current opioid crisis and, in the process, may limit access to pain medications for older adults who need them.[31] Lack of access to providers and medications can contribute to undertreatment as well. These factors are just some of the challenges to effective pain management that may contribute to unrelieved pain among older adults.

Persistent pain and mood symptoms, such as depression, are integrally related, but the direction of the effect is not always clear. Depression may predispose older adults to the experience of pain; pain may be a somatic expression of the depression. Conversely, the experience of living with persistent pain may lead to depressed mood. Regardless of the direction, these 2 phenomena are intertwined. Losses associated with aging may contribute to depressed and anxious mood. These psychosocial conditions may affect older adults' attitudes and beliefs about pain, expectations of pain management, and adherence to pain treatment.[32] Clinicians should assess older adults' social history and psychological state, as these factors may significantly influence the pain experience for older adults.

Consequences of Pain in Older Adults

Despite the recent scientific and clinical attention to pain, evidence suggests that pain management for older adults remains suboptimal across care settings.[12,13,33] Untreated or ineffectively treated moderate to severe persistent pain has significant implications for older adults' health, functioning, and quality of life. Unrelieved pain is associated with impaired physical functioning (impaired mobility, gait disturbances, falls), mental and social functioning (depression, anxiety, social withdrawal, decreased activity engagement).[7] Pain is also associated with sleep disturbances, cognitive decline, malnutrition, and slowed rehabilitation.[7] Pain also increases caregiving burdens for family members who must often assist with treatments to alleviate pain at home.[34] Ultimately, unrelieved pain reduces quality of life for older adults and contributes to increased health care resource utilization and costs.[11,35,36] Thus, it is not surprising that the Institute of Medicine declared chronic pain a public health problem in the United States.[11]

Effective pain management requires comprehensive assessment and treatment. Thus, these 2 components of pain management are discussed separately. The following sections of this article provide an evidence-based approach to the assessment of pain in older adults. The goal is to provide information that can be used to improve the care of older adults experiencing pain.

PAIN ASSESSMENT IN OLDER ADULTS

In clinical settings, health care providers typically assess pain with 2 questions: (1) "Are you having any pain?" and (2) "On a scale of 1 to 10, how much pain are you having?" Those basic questions provide a quick assessment of the presence of pain and its intensity. In 2006, Carl Von Baeyer[37] eloquently stated that "measuring pain by its intensity alone is like describing music only in terms of its loudness." As highlighted in the IASP definition, pain is a multidimensional phenomenon. Thus, comprehensive pain assessment is necessary to ascertain a more complete picture of people's pain experience. It is important to note that there is no objective biological marker or laboratory test for pain, thus pain assessment must reply on patient self-report. In people who cannot verbalize pain, such as those with dementia or communication disorders, pain assessment must reply on observational measures of pain. These approaches to pain assessment are discussed in the following sections.

Self-Reported Pain

Patients' self-report is considered the gold standard for pain assessment.[7] The first principle of pain assessment is to regularly *ask* about the presence of pain.[5] Older adults may need additional time to answer questions, so it is important to allow sufficient time to respond, especially when working with cognitively impaired older adults. It is also important to explore different words that patients may use synonymously with pain, such as discomfort or aching. Use open-ended questions, such as "Tell me about your pain, aches, soreness, or discomfort," to elicit information about pain from older adults.[33]

Comprehensive pain assessment should include the following: concise medical history, identification of chronic conditions, focused physical examination, biopsychosocial assessment, medications (including over-the-counter), and allergies and drug reactions. Assessment should include evaluation of pain features (eg, frequency, intensity, exacerbating and relieving factors), functional impact, and social factors that may influence pain and pain treatment.[25] Reid and colleagues[14] provide a protocol that includes these elements in a comprehensive geriatric pain assessment form.

Evidence-based assessment tools should be used to document pain and monitor responses to pain treatment. Pain intensity can be measured in various ways. Some commonly used tools include the Numerical Rating Scale (NRS), the Verbal Descriptor Scale (VDS), and the Faces Pain Scale (FPS).[25] The NRS is widely used in clinical settings; patients are asked to rate the intensity of their pain on a 0 to 10 scale. The NRS requires the ability to discriminate differences in pain intensity and may be difficult for some older adults to complete. A recent study confirmed that the NRS was a reliable and valid tool for measuring pain in community-residing elders.[38] However, the investigators reported a significantly higher failure rate in completing the NRS among the oldest-old (>81 years; 11.1% failure rate) compared with those in the young-old (61–70 years; 5.5% failure rate) or old (71–80 years; 7.8% failure rate) age groups. This study also reported that the NRS was a reliable measure of pain over time, a key factor in assessing treatment effectiveness and changes in pain ratings over time (reliability coefficient of 0.85, indicating high measurement reliability). There is evidence that older adults prefer a vertical orientation to the NRS scale when it is presented on paper.[33]

The VDS is specifically recommended for use with older adults.[33] This tool measures pain intensity by asking participants to select a word that best describes their present pain (eg, no pain to worst pain imaginable). This measure has been found to be a reliable and valid measure and is reported to be the easiest to complete and the most preferred by older adults.[23,39] The FPS, initially developed to assess pain intensity in children, is often used to measure pain intensity, especially among cognitively impaired older adults. The FPS and the FPS-Revised consists of facial expressions of pain, ranging from the least pain to the most pain possible.[23] Among adults, the FPS is considered more appropriate than other pictorial scales because the cartoon faces are not age-specific, gender-specific, or race-specific. The Geriatric Pain Web page (http://www.geriatricpain.org) provides access to these tools, as well instructions for their use.

For assessing the functional impact of pain, the Brief Pain Inventory is often used.[39] A short, 3-item version of this scale, called the PEG Scale, is recommended for quick assessment of pain interference with activities.[25,40] Using a 0 to 10 scale, this tool measures patients' average pain experienced, pain interference with enjoyment, and pain interference with general activity over the past week. The score (averaging of the 3 domains) can be used to guide the pain management plan.[25]

To learn more about comprehensive pain assessment and measurement, the reader is referred to several excellent clinical guidelines and consensus statements. The American Pain Society issued an interdisciplinary expert consensus statement on assessment of pain in older persons.[8] This document provides a comprehensive review of a pain assessment, including evaluation of measurement tools and recommendations for pain assessment batteries. This review also addresses the assessment of psychological, emotional, and functional factors that are related to pain in older adults, and provides an excellent overview of appropriate measurement tools in these domains as well. More recently, Booker and Herr[41] described a focused pain assessment protocol for older adults and provided guidelines for selecting pain assessment tools.

Observed Pain Indicators

Comprehensive pain assessment also includes the evaluation of objective indicators of pain. Cognitive impairment, common in many older adults, compromises older adults' ability to self-report pain. In patients with dementia and other patients who cannot provide self-report, other assessment approaches must be used to identify the presence of pain. The American Society for Pain Management Nursing consensus statement on assessing pain in nonverbal patients recommends using a hierarchical pain assessment approach.[10] The 4 steps in the process are as follows: (1) attempt to obtain a self-report of pain; (2) look for an underlying cause of pain, such as surgery or a procedure; (3) observe for pain behaviors; and (4) seek input from family and caregivers.[8] If any of these steps are positive, the nurse should assume that pain is present and a trial of analgesics can be initiated. Pain behaviors should be observed before and after the analgesic trial to evaluate if the treatment was effective or if a stronger dose is needed.

Observational techniques for pain assessment focus on behavioral or nonverbal indicators of pain.[8,13,23] Behaviors such as guarded movement, bracing, rubbing the affected area, grimacing, painful noises or words, and restlessness are considered indicators of pain.[7,13] In the acute care setting, vital signs are often considered physiologic indicators of pain. It is important to note, however, that elevated vital signs are not considered a reliable indicator of persistent pain, although they can be indicative of the need for pain assessment.[10,42]

Over the past few decades, there has been a plethora of different observational measurement tools developed to assess behavioral indicators of pain. These tools differ in their content, comprehensiveness, and scoring. Some have been tested empirically and show utility, but many require further psychometric testing of reliability and validity before they can be recommended for widespread use.[42] There is not one behavioral measure of pain that can be universally applied in all settings or with all nonverbal people. However, a recent panel of experts developed a consensus statement for the use of pain behavior assessment tools in nursing homes[4] and recommended use of the Pain Assessment in Advanced Dementia (PAINAD) scale[43] and the Pain Assessment Checklist for Seniors With Severe Dementia.[44]

More recently, the Mobilization-Observation-Behaviour-Intensity-Dementia Pain Scale (MOBID-2) has gained empirical support as a reliable and valid measure of pain behaviors in patients with advanced dementia.[45] Pain behaviors of vocalizations, facial expressions (eg, grimacing), and body movements (eg, defensive positions such as guarding or pushing) are assessed. The MOBID-2 has 2 parts. Part 1 assesses pain related to the musculoskeletal system (the most common cause of pain in older adults) during a set of standardized, guided movements during morning care (5 items). Part 2 assesses pain that might originate from internal organs, head, and skin and is monitored over time (5 items). If a pain behavior is detected, pain intensity is rated by direct caregivers using a 0 to 10 numerical rating scale. The psychometric properties of the MOBID-2 demonstrate high interrater and intrarater and test-retest reliability.[46] Internal consistency reliability was also high, with Cronbach alpha ranging from 0.82 to 0.84.[45] Importantly, the MOBID-2 has demonstrated sensitivity to pain treatment and, to date, is the only behavioral measure to evaluate this important dimension of pain treatment.[47]

The Geriatric Pain Web site (http://www.geriatricpain.org) provides access to some of these behavioral measures. In addition, the Hartford Institute for Geriatric Nursing provides online resources for pain assessment in older adults with dementia (https://consultgeri.org/try-this/dementia/issue-d2), including information on the PAI-NAD tool and an instructional video on how to use it.[48] Several caveats about observational tools must be noted: (1) the presence of these behaviors is suggestive of pain but is not a definitive indicator of pain, and (2) the presence of pain behaviors does not provide information about the intensity of pain.[5] As such, pain behavior tools are important, but should be used as part of a comprehensive pain assessment.

SUMMARY

Pain is a significant problem for older adults that has a potential negative influence on independence, functioning, and quality of life. In the acute care setting, pain can negatively affect healing. Systematic and thorough assessment, however, is a critical first step in appropriately managing pain in older adults. This assessment process can be hampered by many factors. The use of a standardized pain assessment tool is important in measuring pain. It enables health care providers to document their assessment, measure change in pain, evaluate treatment effectiveness, and communicate to other health care providers, the patient, and the family. Pain should be assessed using measures of self-reported pain and pain behaviors. Information from family and caregivers also should be obtained, although these data should be considered supplemental rather than definitive.

REFERENCES

1. Altman D, Frist WH. Medicare and Medicaid at 50 years: perspectives of beneficiaries, health care professionals and institutions, and policy makers. JAMA 2015;314(4):384–95.
2. Federal Interagency Forum on Aging-Related Statistics. Older Americans 2012: key indicators of well-being. Washington (DC): Federal Interagency Forum on Aging-Related Statistics; 2012.
3. Joint Commission on the Accreditation of Healthcare Organization. Accreditation manual for hospitals. Oakbrook Terrace (IL): JCAHO; 2001.
4. Herr K, Bursch H, Ersek M, et al. Use of pain-behavioral assessment tools in the nursing home: expert consensus recommendations for practice. J Gerontol Nurs 2010;36(3):18–29 [quiz: 30–31].
5. Pasero C, McCaffery M. Pain assessment and pharmacologic management. St. Louis (MO): Mosby Elsevier; 2011.
6. AGS Panel on Persistent Pain in Older Persons. The management of persistent pain in older persons. J Am Geriatr Soc 2002;50(6 Suppl):S205–24.
7. American Geriatrics Society Panel on Pharmacological Management of Persistent Pain in Older Persons. Pharmacological management of persistent pain in older persons. J Am Geriatr Soc 2009;57(8):1331–46.

8. Hadjistavropoulos T, Herr K, Turk D, et al. An interdisciplinary expert consensus statement on assessment of pain in older persons. Clin J Pain 2007; 23(Supplement 1):S1–43.
9. Abdulla A, Bone M, Adams N, et al. Evidence-based clinical practice guidelines on management of pain in older people. Age Ageing 2013;42(2):151–3.
10. Herr K, Coyne PJ, Key T, et al. Pain assessment in the nonverbal patient: position statement with clinical practice recommendations. Pain Manag Nurs 2006;7(2): 44–52.
11. Institute of Medicine: Committee on advancing pain Research Care and Education. Relieving pain in America: a blueprint for transforming prevention, care, education, and research. Washington, DC: National Academies Press; 2011.
12. Morrissey MB, Horgas AL, Miller EA, et al. An interdisciplinary look at the potential of policy to improve the health of an aging America: focus on pain. Washington (DC): The Gerontological Society of America; 2014.
13. Horgas AL, Elliott AF, Marsiske M. Pain assessment in persons with dementia: relationship between self-report and behavioral observation. J Am Geriatr Soc 2009;57(1):126–32.
14. Reid MC, Eccleston C, Pillemer K. Management of chronic pain in older adults. BMJ 2015;350:h532.
15. Morrissey MB, Viola D, Shi Q. Relationship between pain and chronic illness among seriously ill older adults: expanding role for palliative social work. J Soc Work End Life Palliat Care 2014;10(1):8–33.
16. Patel KV, Guralnik JM, Dansie EJ, et al. Prevalence and impact of pain among older adults in the United States: findings from the 2011 National Health and Aging Trends Study. Pain 2013;154(12):2649–57.
17. Abdulla A, Adams N, Bone M, et al. Guidance on the management of pain in older people. Age Ageing 2013;42(suppl 1):i1–57.
18. Savvas SM, Gibson SJ. Overview of pain management in older adults. Clin Geriatr Med 2016;32(4):635–50.
19. Anpalahan M, Savvas S, Lo KY, et al. Chronic idiopathic normocytic anaemia in older people: the risk factors and the role of age-associated renal impairment. Aging Clin Exp Res 2017;29(2):147–55.
20. Merskey H. Logic, truth and language in concepts of pain. Qual Life Res 1994; 3(Suppl 1):S69–76.
21. Melzack R, Casey KL. Sensory, motivational, and central control determinants of pain. The skin senses. Springfield (IL): Charles C. Thomas; 1968. p. 423-39.
22. McCaffery M. Nursing practice theories related to cognition, bodily pain and man-environmental interactions. Los Angeles (CA): UCLA Students Store; 1968.
23. Herr K, Bjoro K, Decker S. Tools for assessment of pain in nonverbal older adults with dementia: a state-of-the-science review. J pain symptom Manag 2006;31(2): 170–92.
24. Bruckenthal P, Reid MC, Reisner L. Special issues in the management of chronic pain in older adults. Pain Med 2009;10(Suppl 2):S67–78.
25. Guerriero F, Bolier R, Van Cleave JH, et al. Pharmacological approaches for the management of persistent pain in older adults: what nurses need to know. J Gerontol Nurs 2016;42(12):49–57.
26. Macrae WA. Chronic post-surgical pain: 10 years on. Br J Anaesth 2008;101(1): 77–86.
27. Kehlet H, Jensen TS, Woolf CJ. Persistent postsurgical pain: risk factors and prevention. Lancet 2006;367(9522):1618–25.

28. Lukas A, Barber JB, Johnson P, et al. Observer-rated pain assessment instruments improve both the detection of pain and the evaluation of pain intensity in people with dementia. Eur J Pain 2013;17(10):1558–68.
29. Horgas AL, Tsai PF. Analgesic drug prescription and use in cognitively impaired nursing home residents. Nurs Res 1998;47(4):235–42.
30. Morrison RS, Magaziner J, Gilbert M, et al. Relationship between pain and opioid analgesics on the development of delirium following hip fracture. J Gerontol A Biol Sci Med Sci 2003;58(1):76–81.
31. Guerriero F, Reid MC. New opioid prescribing guidelines released in the US: what impact will they have in the care of older patients with persistent pain? Curr Med Res Opin 2017;33(2):275–8.
32. Reid MC. Expanding targets for intervention in later life pain: what role can patient beliefs, expectations, and pleasant activities play? Clin Geriatr Med 2016;32(4):797–805.
33. Herr K. Pain assessment strategies in older patients. J Pain 2011;12(3 Suppl 1):S3–13.
34. Reinhard S, Levine C, Samis S. Home alone: family caregivers providing complex chronic care. Washington, DC: AARP Public Policy Institute; 2012.
35. Griffin DW, Harmon D, Kennedy N. Do patients with chronic low back pain have an altered level and/or pattern of physical activity compared to healthy individuals? A systematic review of the literature. Physiotherapy 2012;98(1):13–23.
36. Johansen A, Romundstad L, Nielsen CS, et al. Persistent postsurgical pain in a general population: prevalence and predictors in the Tromsø study. Pain 2012;153(7):1390–6.
37. von Baeyer CL. Children's self-reports of pain intensity: scale selection, limitations and interpretation. Pain Res Manag 2006;11(3):157–62.
38. Wood BM, Nicholas MK, Blyth F, et al. Assessing pain in older people with persistent pain: the NRS is valid but only provides part of the picture. J Pain 2010;11(12):1259–66.
39. Cleeland CS, Ryan KM. Pain assessment: global use of the brief pain inventory. Ann Acadmed Singapore 1994;23(2):129–38.
40. Krebs EE, Lorenz KA, Bair MJ, et al. Development and initial validation of the PEG, a three-item scale assessing pain intensity and interference. J Gen Intern Med 2009;24(6):733–8.
41. Booker SQ, Herr KA. Assessment and measurement of pain in adults in later life. Clin Geriatr Med 2016;32(4):677–92.
42. Herr K, Coyne PJ, McCaffery M, et al. Pain assessment in the patient unable to self-report: position statement with clinical practice recommendations. Pain Manag Nurs 2011;12(4):230–50.
43. Warden V, Hurley AC, Volicer L. Development and psychometric evaluation of the Pain Assessment in Advanced Dementia (PAINAD) scale. J Am Med Dir Assoc 2003;4(1):9–15.
44. Fuchs-Lacelle S, Hadjistavropoulos T. Development and preliminary validation of the pain assessment checklist for seniors with limited ability to communicate (PACSLAC). Pain Manag Nurs 2004;5(1):37–49.
45. Husebo BS, Strand LI, Moe-Nilssen R, et al. Pain in older persons with severe dementia. Psychometric properties of the Mobilization-Observation-Behaviour-Intensity-Dementia (MOBID-2) Pain Scale in a clinical setting. Scand J Caring Sci 2010;24(2):380–91.

46. Sandvik RK, Selbaek G, Seifert R, et al. Impact of a stepwise protocol for treating pain on pain intensity in nursing home patients with dementia: a cluster randomized trial. Eur J Pain 2014;18(10):1490–500.
47. Husebo BS, Ostelo R, Strand LI. The MOBID-2 pain scale: reliability and responsiveness to pain in patients with dementia. Eur J Pain 2014;18(10):1419–30.
48. Horgas A, Miller L. Pain assessment in people with dementia. Am J Nurs 2008; 108(7):62–70 [quiz: 71].

Impaired Sleep
A Multifaceted Geriatric Syndrome

Grace E. Dean, PhD, RN[a],*, Carleara Weiss, PhD, RN[a],
Jonna L. Morris, BSN, RN[b], Eileen R. Chasens, PhD, RN[b]

KEYWORDS

• Geriatric syndrome • Circadian rhythms • Sleep

KEY POINTS

General:
• Normal sleep changes and impaired sleep accompany the aging process.
• Common sleep disorders in older adults are addressed, with information regarding treatments that can both help and hurt sleep.

More specific:
• Hospitalized older adults are vulnerable to impaired sleep, which can contribute to delirium and delayed healing.

IMPAIRED SLEEP AS A GERIATRIC SYNDROME

When older adults complain that they "didn't sleep well" or they "wake up when it is still night time," they are not describing a specific disease. The older adult may be describing a geriatric syndrome that results from multiple risk factors that collectively cause impaired nighttime sleep or a disrupted circadian rhythm pattern. Impaired nighttime sleep can result in excessive daytime sleepiness, decreased daytime function, and reduced physical, psychological, and social well-being. Most seriously, impaired sleep is also implicated in potentially life-threatening events such as a fall on the way to the bathroom because of nocturia or development of delirium during hospitalization. This article explains why impaired sleep in older adults is considered a geriatric syndrome, explains the effect of normal aging on sleep, and describes the multiple diseases, medications, and other reasons that can negatively affect sleep.

Disclosure Statement: There are no commercial or financial conflicts of interest for all authors.
[a] Department of Biobehavioral Health and Clinical Sciences, School of Nursing, University at Buffalo, 3435 Main Street, 301 Wende Hall, Buffalo, NY 14214, USA; [b] Department of Health and Community Systems, School of Nursing, University of Pittsburgh, 415 Victoria Building, 3500 Victoria Street, Pittsburgh, PA 15261, USA
* Corresponding author.
E-mail address: gdean@buffalo.edu

One fact that must be recognized is that impaired sleep is not part of normal aging; it is dangerous for either patients or clinicians to consider that poor sleep is a normal or expected condition for older adults.

Although the term "older adults" refers to persons 65 years of age or older, it is important to recognize that persons who are very old (ie, 85 years old and older) are at the greatest risk for geriatric syndromes. The term "geriatric syndrome" refers to when there is a clinical condition that has multiple possible causes or does not have a clearly defined cause of a single distinct disease; for example, frailty or delirium that results in negative outcomes.[1] Impaired sleep in older adults shares many features with other geriatric syndromes because it frequently (1) increases in prevalence in older adults, (2) has symptoms and outcomes that differ from the underlying pathologies or precipitating causes, (3) may have multiple causative factors, and (4) too frequently results in a downward trajectory of decreased health or well-being.[1,2]

The importance of sleep and circadian rhythms on healthy aging was the focus of a recent American Geriatrics Society/National Institute of Aging conference. Experts described how impaired sleep and circadian rhythms negatively affect older adults' brain health, physical health, and functional status and then proposed a research agenda to address gaps in the knowledge.[3] Nurse-clinicians and researchers need to remember that impaired sleep in older adults may deteriorate into a geriatric syndrome that is characterized by detrimental changes in sleep in older adults.

Older adults are at high risk for geriatric sleep syndrome because not only do they have a normal change in the sleep-wake processes that occurs with aging, but they also have the following: (1) increased risk for many sleep disorders, (2) increased use of medications that are associated with either oversedation and/or excessive sleepiness or, conversely, hypervigilance and insomnia, (3) an increased prevalence in chronic diseases that may negatively impact sleep, (4) increased risk for hospitalization's effects on sleep, (5) symptoms such as pain and nocturia, and (6) changes in social roles such as caregiving, widowhood, or retirement that may negatively impact sleep. The purpose of this review is to describe each of these factors and how these factors may interact with each other to result in negative outcomes. Finally, the review suggests interventions and collaborations that the nurse can use to help prevent the downward spiral of events that can occur from impaired sleep and to promote healthy sleep in older adults.

NORMAL CHANGES IN SLEEP WITH AGING
Normal Sleep

Sleep is a fundamental physiologic process that is as essential to life as is breathing or eating. Sleep is often thought of as a time of rest and recovery from the challenges of everyday life. However, research is revealing that sleep is a complicated state involving behavioral and physiologic processes. Sleep plays an important role in many aspects of health and disease, including metabolism,[4] cardiovascular disease,[5] quality of life,[6] and even caregiver burden.[7] The consequences of insufficient sleep on neurobehavioral and cognitive functioning, such as deficits in sustained attention, reaction time, working memory, and executive functioning, are well documented.[8]

Normal human sleep is divided into 2 phases: non–rapid eye movement (NREM) sleep and rapid eye movement (REM) sleep. NREM sleep is further categorized into 3 stages (N1, N2, and N3) identified through unique electroencephalographic and electromyelographic waveforms and frequencies. N3, also known as slow-wave sleep, correlates with the release of growth hormone. A sleep cycle consists of the progression through the 3 NREM stages (N1–N3), ending in REM sleep encompassing 70 to 120 minutes per cycle. Typically, 4 to 6 cycles of NREM-REM sleep occur per night. The gradual decline in slow-wave sleep starts during adolescence and continues to decline throughout the lifespan, plateauing at approximately age 60.[9]

Sleep in Older Adults

Normal aging is associated with changes in sleep architecture. Older adults are at risk for age-related sleep changes that include increased sleep onset latency and wake after sleep onset (WASO), a reduction in slow-wave and REM sleep, and advanced sleep phase syndrome.[10–12] Age-related changes are associated with changes in the neural sleep circuitry; a decline in central nervous system endogenous neuropeptides orexin A and B, also called hypocretin 1 and 2, and expression levels with aging have been observed.[13] Normally, hypocretins are active during wakefulness and silent during sleep.[14] Results of these sleep changes can lead to less total sleep time, poorer sleep efficiency, and increased daytime napping.[15] Excessive daytime sleepiness is not part of normal aging and needs to be evaluated.[16]

Age-related changes are noticeable in circadian rhythms[17] that are controlled by a master clock, the suprachiasmatic nuclei (SCN), located deep within the brain.[18] The SCN regulates sleep-wake patterns, hormone secretion, and cognitive performance using environmental cues to entrain these rhythms to an approximately 24-hour cycle.[19] The light-dark cycle is the strongest environmental cue for circadian entrainment.[19]

The normal aging process affects brain structures, such as frontal cortical areas, hypothalamus (where the SCN is located), and the brainstem locus coeruleus.[20] As a consequence of these changes, the SCN's ability to maintain a stable circadian rhythm is reduced with age.[20] Furthermore, with advancing age, there is a decline in the cortisol and melatonin rhythms.[21] In addition, aging reduces sensitivity to light at the retinal level which also contributes to circadian disruptions in older adults[22] because light at the retinal level is crucial for the circadian entrainment via the nonvisual pathway that communicates light from the eyes to the SCN.

COMMON SLEEP DISORDERS IN OLDER ADULTS
Insomnia

Insomnia is the most common sleep disturbance reported by healthy adults with a prevalence rate of 20% to 40% for insomnia symptoms versus 5% for an insomnia diagnosis across all adult age groups.[23] Prevalence for older adults was 21% in those 65 years of age and older.[23] Insomnia is characterized by repeated difficulty falling asleep, difficulty staying asleep, early morning awakening, and daytime sleepiness that negatively impacts functioning despite adequate time and opportunity for sleep that occurs at least 3 times per week for more than 1 month.[24] Short sleepers, less than 6 hours a night, are distinguished from those with true insomnia by the added complaint of daytime dysfunction.

Risk factors for the development of insomnia are discussed using the Spielman 3-factor model that identifies predisposing, precipitating, and perpetuating factors.[25] Predisposing factors include genetic variants in clock genes, individuals who are female, divorced, separated, or widowed, and those with lower levels of education.[26] Life stressors, medical or psychiatric illnesses, or treatments for these conditions constitute precipitating factors. Perpetuating factors are behavioral or cognitive changes that result in the persistence of the acute insomnia, leading to chronicity.

Untreated insomnia in the older adult can lead to an increased risk for the development of depression, heart disease, cancer, and cognitive impairment.[27–30] Remarkably, one study examining objective sleep fragmentation revealed that participants in the highest 10% of sleep fragmentation had a 50% increased risk of developing Alzheimer disease compared with those in the lowest 10%.[31] Quality of life is often worse in older adults with insomnia.[32]

Cognitive behavioral therapy (CBT) interventions are thought to affect symptoms by changing symptom-related thoughts, diminishing beliefs that exacerbate symptoms, and increasing personal perceptions of control over symptoms; it is as effective as pharmacologic treatments in patients with insomnia without the added side effects or relapses seen with drug treatment.[33,34]

Sleep-Disordered Breathing

Sleep-disordered breathing (SDB) refers to events during sleep that result in decreased or cessation of breathing. Included are obstructive sleep apnea (OSA) and central sleep apnea. OSA occurs when there is a narrowing or collapse of the pharyngeal airway that results in repeated hypopneas (reduction in airflow to <50% of normal that is accompanied by an oxygen desaturation) and apneas (cessation of airflow) that last for at least 10 seconds while there is continued respiratory effort. Central sleep apnea occurs when the brain fails to signal the need for respiration that results in apneas without continued respiratory effort. In addition, there are "mixed apneas" that may start as an obstructive apnea or hypopnea that progresses to a central apnea, or vice versa.[35] Apneas and hypopneas are stopped when low oxygen saturation results in a brief arousal (<10 seconds) and resumption of breathing. Severity of SDB is defined according to the apnea + hypopnea index (AHI), the average number of hourly events, and described as "mild" (AHI = 5–14), "moderate" (AHI = 15–29), and "severe" (AHI ≥30).[35]

A landmark epidemiologic study estimated the prevalence of SDB in 30- to 60-year-old adults to be 4% of men and 2% of women.[36] The prevalence of SDB in older adults is much higher. A review of studies of older adults estimated the prevalence as 13% to 32%.[37] Risk factors for OSA in older adults are somewhat different than those in younger adults; although obesity and male gender remain risk factors, older adults frequently are less obese or overweight compared with younger adults, and the risk for women by age 50 approaches that of men.[38] Several studies suggest that older adults have an increased risk for OSA because of decreased airway stability that is associated with age-related changes in the anatomic structure of the upper airway and to decreased neuromuscular response to negative pressure or hypoxia.[39,40] Increased prevalence of central sleep apnea among older adults may be secondary to the increased prevalence of comorbidities such as heart failure where half of the patient's SDB is frequently dominated by central apneas and Cheyne-Stokes respirations.[41] Negative outcomes for older adults with SDB include excessive daytime sleepiness, cognitive dysfunction, and an increased risk of cardiovascular morbidity and mortality.[37]

The nurse can assess for SDB by asking older adults if anyone tells them that they snore, wake up with a gasp or "snorting noise," or observed pauses in their breathing during sleep.[42] Many older adults sleep without a bed partner who can detect symptoms of SDB. If the persons are at high risk or with symptoms of SDB, they should be referred to their primary care provider for further evaluation. Diagnosis of SDB is determined with a home or in-laboratory–based polysomnography sleep study. Treatment of SDB is similar to that used in younger persons; the "gold standard" for treatment of OSA is continuous positive airway pressure (CPAP). The use of oral appliances may be appropriate if the older adult has stable dentition. Treatment of central sleep apnea–dominant SDB or mixed apnea requires not only evaluation of the pattern of apneas but also whether the older adult has coexisting heart failure; it may involve use of bile-vel CPAP that includes pressure support for treatment of central apneas.

Restless Legs Syndrome

Restless legs syndrome (RLS), also known as Willis-Ekbom disease, is highly prevalent among persons older than 65 years, with an estimated prevalence of 10% to 35%.[43] The diagnosis of RLS depends on 5 clinical criteria being met, accompanied by an urge to move legs that (1) is accompanied by uncomfortable sensations, (2) increases during rest or inactivity, (3) is relieved or reduced by movement, (4) increases in severity in the evening or night, and (5) is not explained by other medical conditions.[44] Periodic limb movements that occur during sleep result in arousals and sleep fragmentation that are associated with excessive daytime sleepiness. Sleep problems associated with RLS include insomnia with the decreased ability to initiate and maintain sleep. Risk factors in older adults for RLS include peripheral neuropathy, iron-deficiency anemia, and uremia secondary to renal failure. Initial treatment of RLS usually includes correction of these risk factors and lifestyle modifications, such as avoiding caffeine, cigarettes, and alcohol, maintaining a regular sleep schedule, and mild to moderate exercise. Medications used to treat RLS include pergolide, prami-pexole, ropinirole, and levodopa/carbidopa; 2 anticonvulsant medications, gabapentin and carbamazepine, are prescribed for painful symptoms.[43]

Rapid Eye Movement Behavior Disorder

Normally, during REM sleep there is paralysis (atonia) of the skeletal muscles that prevents physically acting out dreams while sleeping. In REM behavior disorder (RBD), this is missing. RBD is primarily found in men, usually beginning between ages 40 and 70,[45] and the estimated prevalence is 0.5%.[46] Many times the sleeper will remember the dreams as nightmares.[45] The sleeper may kick, punch, shout, jump, or act out any other scenarios of a dream. The bed partner can be injured as a result of RBD. The activity occurs during the REM stages of sleep, particularly in the hours just before wakening. RBD may appear in clusters happening several nights in a row and then not at all for months.[45] Increased prevalence of RBD is associated with Parkinson disease, Alzheimer disease, Lewy body dementia, multiple system atrophy, and other neurodegenerative disorders, but is not always indicative of one of these disorders.[45] Certain medications such as selective serotonin reuptake inhibitors (SSRIs) and selective noradrenergic reuptake inhibitors have also been implicated. RBD is diagnosed using polysomnography with video monitoring because OSA may also cause similar symptoms.[45] Treatment of RBD involves managing the dreams and their resulting behaviors. In patients without OSA or cognitive impairment, medications such as clonazepam and melatonin have been found to be effective. It is also necessary to protect both the patient and the bed partner from harm.[45]

Circadian Rhythm Disorders

Current evidence posits that circadian rhythm disorders are the leading cause of sleep problems in older adults, with sleep phase advancement being the most common.[47] Described as typical early sleep times (6-9 PM) and early wake up (2-5 AM),[48] individuals often complain about insomnia, early morning awakening, followed by daytime sleepiness especially in the late afternoon or early evening.[49] Diminished retinal response to morning light exposure may also contribute to advanced sleep phase disorder (ASPD) in older adults.[48] Other circadian disorders include irregular sleep-wake sleep disorder and non-24-hour sleep-wake type.[22]

MEDICATIONS AND SLEEP

In 2005, the National Institutes of Health State of the Science Conference focused on chronic insomnia in adults and reported that the only support for pharmacologic treatment of insomnia was with the use of benzodiazepine receptor agonists.[50] **Table 1** describes the US Food and Drug Administration (FDA)-approved benzodiazepine receptor agonists for insomnia management, which include benzodiazepines, nonbenzodiazepines, and ramelteon, a melatonin receptor agonist, and several other commonly used medications. According to the American Geriatric Society, the use of many of these medications is to be avoided.

Benzodiazepines have been shown to have positive effects on sleep latency, total sleep time, and WASO in clinical trials involving non–cancer insomniacs.[51] Long-acting benzodiazepines may result in adverse effects, such as residual sedation, undesired behaviors during sleep, falls, and memory and performance impairment. Nonbenzodiazepine pharmaceuticals have shorter active metabolic half-lives and as a result are less associated with daytime impairments.[52] These prescribed medications provide short-term relief, but their efficacy has not been demonstrated beyond 12 weeks.[53] Sleep clinicians often recommend a 1-month trial because of the lack of long-term efficacy data and the potential issues with rebound insomnia and withdrawal. Regardless, short-term hypnotic treatment should be supplemented with behavioral and cognitive therapies whenever possible.

Use of hypnotic medications in older adults should be those with a short half-life, at the lowest dose, and avoided because of problems with excessive sedation and increased risk for falls.[54] Importantly, use of hypnotic medications is not advised in persons with untreated SDB because of the potential for further depression of nocturnal respiration. Older adults are frequently on multiple medications that can cause either oversedation that is especially problematic for persons with SDB, or hypervigilance that exacerbates insomnia. **Table 2** lists medications for medical disorders that older adults are frequently prescribed that may affect sleep. "Lifestyle" drugs, such as alcohol, caffeine, and nicotine, frequently affect nighttime sleep. Although alcohol decreases sleep latency so that persons fall asleep more quickly, alcohol use disrupts REM sleep and prevents deep slow-wave sleep. Caffeine (coffee, NoDoz) and nicotine (cigarettes, chewing tobacco, vapes) are stimulants and result in difficulty initiating sleep, restlessness, irritability, headache, lighter sleep, and frequent nighttime awakenings. Finally, although older adults may think herbal medications for sleep such as melatonin and valerian are "natural" and therefore safer, these substances are not FDA regulated and there are insufficient data on their safety in older adults.[52]

MEDICAL CONDITIONS THAT AFFECT SLEEP

Although normal age is not synonymous with diseases, the prevalence of chronic illnesses increases with aging. Many diseases and the medications that are used to treat them can both be associated with increased risk for sleep disorders and the negative effects of disrupted sleep on management of the medical disorder. A partial list of medical conditions that are associated with impaired sleep in older adults includes cardiovascular disease,[12,55–62] diabetes,[63–66] cancer,[67–69] chronic obstructive pulmonary disease,[70] and immune diseases such as rheumatic arthritis.[71]

SLEEP AND COGNITIVE IMPAIRMENT

Circadian disruptions observed may be connected to mood, cognition, and neurodegenerative disorders in older adults. First, delay or advance in circadian timing

Table 1
Sleep medications, adverse effects, and implications for older adults

Medications That Effect Sleep	Used to Treat	Examples	Adverse Effects	Implications for Older Adults
Nonbenzodiazepine receptor agonists	Sleep-onset latency Sleep maintenance Nighttime awakening	Eszopiclone, Zaleplon, Zolpidem	Headache, dizziness, gastrointestinal disturbances, daytime sleepiness Zolpidem additionally: amnesia, hallucinations, unusual nighttime behaviors	Avoid, minimal improvement on sleep latency, increased risk of a patient fall
Benzodiazepines	Sleep-onset latency Sleep maintenance Nighttime awakening	Triazolam, Estazolam, Flurazepam, Temazepam	Daytime sleepiness, dizziness, fall risk, mobility problems	Avoid, increased risk of oversedation with cognitive impairment, delirium, and risk of falls
Melatonin receptor agonists	Sleep-onset latency	Ramelteon	Headache, daytime sleepiness	
Antidepressants	Sleep-onset latency Sleep maintenance Nighttime awakening	Mirtazapine, Doxepin, Trazodone	Headache, daytime sleepiness, anticholinergic effects	If indicated for depression, administration at bedtime will reduce sedative effectives
Over the counter	Sleep-onset latency	Diphenhydramine	Daytime sleepiness, anticholinergic effects	Avoid, increased risk of oversedation with cognitive impairment, delirium, and risk of falls
Herbal	Sleep-onset latency	Melatonin, Valerian	Headache, daytime sleepiness, depression	Not FDA regulated

Data from Schroeck JL, Ford J, Conway EL, et al. Review of safety and efficacy of sleep medicines in older adults. Clin Ther 2016;38(11):2340–72; and American Geriatrics Society 2015 Beers Criteria Update Expert Panel. American Geriatrics Society 2015 updated beers criteria for potentially inappropriate medication use in older adults. J Am Geriatr Soc 2015;63(11):2227–46.

Table 2
Medications that can impair sleep

Medication	Indication	Example	Negative Effects
Angiotensin-converting enzyme inhibitors	High blood pressure	Diphenhydramine (Benadryl) Lisinopril (Zestril)	Nighttime cough
Alpha-blockers (alpha-adrenergic antagonists)	High blood pressure, benign prostatic hyperplasia	Doxazosin (Cadura) Prazosin (Minipress) Terazosin (Hytrin)	Headache Pounding heartbeat Weakness Dizziness Weight gain
Beta-blockers	High blood pressure	Atenolol (Tenormin) Metoprolol (Lopressor, Tropol) Propranolol (Inderal)	Insomnia, nightmares
Antihistamines	Allergies / Motion sickness	Diphenhydramine (Benadryl), NyQuil Dimenhydrinate (Dramamine)	Daytime sleepiness, drowsiness
Antipsychotics	Schizophrenia, bipolar disorder	Trazadone (Desyrel) Risperidone (Risperdal) Haloperidol (Haldol)	Daytime sleepiness and sedation
Benzodiazepines	Anxiety	Alprazolam (Xanax), Lorazepam (Ativan)	Respiratory depression, hypoxemia
Corticosteroids	Asthma, chronic obstructive pulmonary disease	Methylprednisolone (Medrol), prednisone	Difficulty falling and staying asleep, abnormal dreams
Opioids	Pain	Morphine, Oxycodone (OxyContin)	Reduction of slow-wave sleep, daytime fatigue, respiratory depression, hypoxemia
SSRIs	Depression, anxiety	Citalopram (Celexa), Escitalopram (Lexapro), Fluoxetine (Prozac)	Restless leg syndrome, insomnia, daytime sleepiness, decreased REM sleep
Sympathomimetic stimulants	Attention deficit	Dextroamphetamine (Adderall) Methamphetamine Methylphenidate (Ritalin)	Decreased REM and non-REM deep sleep Increase sleep onset latency
Tricyclic antidepressants	Depression	Amitriptyline (Elavil), Amoxapine (Asendin), Clomipramine (Anafranil)	Morning grogginess, insomnia, daytime sleepiness, RLS

Data from Refs.[108–111]

combined with damped circadian function is associated with depression in older adults.[72] Second, evidence shows sleep and circadian function impact cognitive performance and alertness[17] and are associated with cognitive decline and neurodegeneration.[73,74] Furthermore, changes in the sleep-wake cycle that accompany geriatric syndromes are associated with a deficit in memory, psychomotor vigilance, and over-all decline in cognitive function.[74] Last, aging-related changes in brain structures, such as frontal cortical areas, hypothalamus, basal forebrain, and brainstem, contribute to circadian disruptions in older adults[17] and may be a predictor of neurodegenerative disorders such as Alzheimer and Parkinson.[74] Recent evidence suggests that fragmented circadian rhythms are common early signs of Alzheimer and Parkinson; these symptoms get worse as the illness progresses.[74]

Effect of Depression, Pain, and Nocturia on Sleep in Older Adults

Depression

Although late-life depression is not part of normal aging, data suggest there is an association between poor sleep and depression in older adults. Some studies identify depression as a risk factor for sleep difficulty, whereas others identify sleep problems as a symptom of depression.[75,76] A meta-analysis investigating subjective sleep quality and depression in the elderly identified a significant relationship in older adults.[76] Poor sleep quality, low sleep efficiency, increased sleep latency, and daytime sleepiness are all reported by depressed older adults.[75]

Treatment of depression includes pharmacologic and nonpharmacologic interventions such as antidepressants and CBT. CBT may be a good option for the treatment of depression in older adults, collaborating to diminish insomnia-like symptoms such as difficulty initiating sleep, difficulty maintaining sleep, and early wakening. The effectiveness depends on factors such as the individuals' cognitive performance and number of CBT sessions.[23]

Pain

Many older adults suffer chronic pain, especially women and those people older than 85 years.[77] Osteoarthritis, a common cause of chronic pain in older adults, is associated with impaired sleep.[78] In order for nurses to help patients get restorative sleep, it is imperative to treat the patient's pain. Recent research suggests that pain does not impair sleep so much as impaired sleep predicts incidences of chronic pain.[79] Short sleep duration or deprivation has been shown to increase pain sensitivity.[79] Studies of sleep architecture show that sleep disturbances may in fact inhibit the processes that mitigate pain. As a result, nonrestorative sleep may be an important predictor of widespread pain in older adults.[80] In addition, as many as 50% of people with insomnia, many of whom are older adults, suffer from chronic pain.[81] Therefore, not only is it important to treat nighttime pain in the older adult, but also it may be even more important to ensure they get restful restorative sleep in order to mitigate their pain throughout the day.

Several factors may affect the relationship of sleep and pain in older adults. Long-term use of opioids can disturb sleep architecture, leading to impaired sleep and thus increased pain. Negative mood and pain catastrophizing can worsen symptoms. African Americans and women have worse sleep quality and more sensitivity to pain than whites and men.[79]

In summary, although it is important to treat nighttime pain, nurses should also take into account impaired sleep as an additional source of increased pain. Before pharmacologic interventions, nurses may want to consider several options to help patients experiencing chronic pain to have better sleep.

Nocturia

Nocturia, waking to void one or more times per night, is a common problem in older adults; as many as 60% of older adults void 2 or more times per night.[82] Voiding more than 2 or more times per night is associated with many comorbidities, including, but not limited to, high blood pressure, diabetes, arthritis, asthma, heart disease, anxiety, depression, benign prostatic hyperplasia, and inflammatory bowel disease.[83] Nocturia can result from increased nocturnal urine production in persons with OSA.[84] In addition, nocturia can impact the quality of life by leading to insomnia from the fragmented sleep and to difficulty in returning to sleep after awakening. People with nocturia are less active the next day.[85] A fall because of rushing to the bathroom significantly increases the risk for mortality.[86]

Changes in Social Roles and Sleep

Caregiving

Older caregivers are at higher risk for age-related sleep changes, sleep disorders such as insomnia, and inadequate sleep duration; women report higher rates of insomnia than men.[87] Evidence suggests that caregiving stress increases vulnerability to chronic disease.[88] Insufficient sleep and daytime fatigue may result in perpetuating compensatory habits, such as daytime napping, spending time in bed not sleeping, and/or avoiding the bed (ie, sleeping on the couch).

Caregivers are at risk for chronic sleep loss. Consequences of chronic sleep loss are well known and include metabolic and inflammatory changes that lead to glucose intolerance and insulin sensitivity, weight gain, cardiovascular disease, and premature death.[12,64,67] Studies have shown that CBT, relaxation, and mindfulness training can improve caregiver mood and sleep quality.[89,90]

Widowhood and retirement

There is limited research regarding sleep problems related to family and socioeconomic characteristics in older adults.[91–93] A European survey, involving 54,722 respondents from 16 countries, assessed health conditions during widowhood and retirement identified that sleep problems bother older adults for at least 6 months[93] Overall prevalence for sleep problems was 24% for the total European sample, but varied between countries from a low of 16.6% in Denmark and Italy to a high of 31.2% in Poland. Consistent with previous literature, women were more likely to report sleep problems than men.[91] Marital status revealed that those who were separated, divorced, or widowed were more likely to report sleep problems.[93] Higher education and household income were associated with less sleep problems.[93] Only those permanently sick or disabled had more sleep problems than retired individuals.[93] These results highlight that family and sociocultural changes and problems can affect sleep in older adults.

SLEEP IN THE HOSPITAL ENVIRONMENT

Noise, patient care interactions, and mechanical ventilation can cause sleep disruption in the hospitalized older patient.[94] The hospital environment is noisy, with average decibel volumes twice what is recommended.[95,96] Noise is responsible for as many as 17% of nighttime arousals in the hospital.[97] Nurses may perform patient care in the intensive care units (ICUs) on the nightshift, contributing to fragmented sleep. In addition, although medically necessary, mechanical ventilation is known to disrupt sleep. Patient factors such as pain, anxiety, medications, and previous co-morbidities such as obstructive sleep merge with the hospital environment to impair sleep.[94]

Sleep deprivation in the acutely ill ICU patient may lead to the onset of delirium.[98] Impaired sleep leads to reduced activity and energy levels,[99] which contribute to a longer recovery process. In order to promote healthy sleep in older hospitalized patients, staff needs to evaluate their routines to minimize sleep interruption and to decrease noise at night.

NONPHARMACOLOGIC APPROACHES TO IMPROVE SLEEP IN OLDER ADULTS

Nonpharmacologic approaches to sleep include sleep hygiene,[100] cognitive behavioral treatment,[27] bright light treatment,[20] exercise,[101] and mind-body activities such as yoga[102] and tai chi.[103] These interventions may be used instead of or in conjunction with medications or other treatments to improve sleep. Nonpharmacologic treatments have the benefit that there is no risk of medication side effect or reaction.

Sleep Hygiene

Good sleep hygiene refers to engaging in behaviors that will promote sleep. Sleep patterns are a learned behavior, and establishing healthy behaviors is foundational to healthy sleep and circadian rhythms in older adults. These behaviors are a good topic to review with patients to see if there are activities that could be modified to improve sleep. Simple sleep hygiene includes maintaining a regular bedtime and wakeup time, avoiding caffeinated foods, beverages, and nicotine, and making the sleep environment inviting with the bedroom dark, quiet, and a comfortable temperature. Additional sleep hygiene measures include avoiding alcohol as a sleep medication, obtaining moderate exercise, and having a light bedtime snack if hungry.[100]

Cognitive Behavioral Treatment

Cognitive behavioral therapy for insomnia (CBTi) has been used in a variety of populations to improve insomnia. Shortened versions of CBTi using brief behavioral interventions (BBTi) and therapy phone calls have achieved significant improvements. The benefits of CBTi in older adults include reduced WASO and improved sleep efficiency.[27] Behavioral sleep interventions for both CBTi and BBTi include sleep hygiene, stimulus control, and relaxation skills. Up to 8 sessions are conducted and can be one-on-one, group, by phone call, or even online. The choice of the best type of session for an older adult should include assessing for individual levels of independence and cognitive functioning.

Bright Light Therapy

Manipulations of circadian timing with exposure to natural daylight or bright light therapy is a valuable treatment option to alleviate age-related issues with sleep, daytime alertness,[20] and mood disorders such as depression.[104] In considering circadian rhythm sleep disorders, the American Academy of Sleep Medicine recommends morning bright light therapy for the treatment of delayed sleep phase disorder.[22] The recommendations for ASPD include a planned sleep-wake schedule along with early evening bright light therapy. Education to avoid exposure to bright light in the morning may be part of the treatment.

Mind-Body

Mind-body interventions involve communication from the mind to influence the body and its physiologic responses to maintain or improve health and well-being. Examples of mind-body interventions for improving sleep in older adults include yoga and tai chi. Although more than a series of poses and stretching techniques to improve flexibility, regular yoga practice may provide benefits for healthy older adults. These benefits include better sleep quality, less disturbed sleep, shorten sleep latency, and improved daytime function in healthy older adults.[102] Evidence shows that yoga diminished the need for sleep medication.[102] The benefits of yoga may be associated with the stretching and relaxing muscle exercises along with the breathing exercises.[102] Tai chi, a Chinese exercise that began as a martial art form, involves a series of coordinated sequential movements with a meditational component.[105] The results of one systematic review reported the safety, absence of adverse events, and moderate to high efficacy for sleep quality using tai chi in older adults with sleep problems.[103] Older adults with geriatric syndrome may also potentially benefit from yoga and tai chi depending on their level of independence and physical ability.

Exercise

In community-dwelling older adults, evidence suggests that physical activity is positively associated with sleep duration and might be an effective way of improving sleep quality in depressed older adults.[101] The research suggests that moderate to vigorous physical activity improves sleep quality and executive functioning in older adults, whereas light-intensity physical activity has no significant effects.[106] A large survey of greater than 8000 participants found that the risk of insomnia is lower among individuals that engage in social or physical activities such as walking.[107]

SUMMARY

Older adults are at risk for geriatric sleep syndromes because of the collective effect of the normal decline in sleep and additive impact of multiple risk factors. Not only is there an increased risk for sleep disorders along with increased physical and mental conditions in older adults, but also there is the effect of polypharmacy, including many medications that are associated with decreased cognition, delirium, and falls. Finally, sleep in older adults is negatively affected by the increased prevalence of symptoms such as pain and nocturia, acute disturbances such as hospitalization, and changes in social roles that normally stabilize the sleep/wake pattern. Older adults are especially vulnerable to the effect of geriatric sleep syndrome, with negative effects ranging from worsening of chronic diseases, decreased daytime function, and impaired mood. In addition, older adults are especially at risk for a rapid decline in function if a fall occurs secondary to a failed attempt to reach the bathroom during the night or the development of delirium. Nurses should both assess sleep in older adults and collaborate with other geriatric team members on interventions to improve sleep in their clients.

REFERENCES

1. Inouye SK, Studenski S, Tinetti ME, et al. Geriatric syndromes: clinical, research, and policy implications of a core geriatric concept. J Am Geriatr Soc 2007;55(5): 780–91.
2. Tinetti ME, Fried T. The end of the disease era. Am J Med 2004;116(3):179–85.
3. Fung CH, Vitiello MV, Alessi CA, et al, AGS/NIA Sleep Conference Planning Committee and Faculty. Report and research agenda of the American Geriatrics Society and National Institute on Aging Bedside-to-Bench Conference on Sleep, Circadian Rhythms, and Aging: new avenues for improving brain health, physical health, and functioning. J Am Geriatr Soc 2016;64(12):e238–47.
4. Kim TW, Jeong J-H, Hong S-C. The impact of sleep and circadian disturbance on hormones and metabolism. Int J Endocrinol 2015;2015:591729.

5. Solarz DE, Mullington JM, Meier-Ewert HK. Sleep, inflammation and cardiovascular disease. Front Biosci 2012;4:2490–501.
6. Reid KJ, Martinovich Z, Finkel S, et al. Sleep: a marker of physical and mental health in the elderly. Am J Geriatr Psychiatry 2006;14(10):860–6.
7. McCurry SM, Song Y, Martin JL. Sleep in caregivers: what we know and what we need to learn. Curr Opin Psychiatry 2015;28(6):497–503.
8. Durmer JS, Dinges DF. Neurocognitive consequences of sleep deprivation. Semin Neurol 2005;25(1):117–29.
9. Ohayon MM, Carskadon MA, Guilleminault C, et al. Meta-analysis of quantitative sleep parameters from childhood to old age in healthy individuals: developing normative sleep values across the human lifespan. Sleep 2004;27(7):1255–73.
10. Huang YL, Liu RY, Wang QS, et al. Age-associated difference in circadian sleep-wake and rest-activity rhythms. Physiol Behav 2002;76(4–5):597–603.
11. Moraes W, Piovezan R, Poyares D, et al. Effects of aging on sleep structure throughout adulthood: a population-based study. Sleep Med 2014;15(4):401–9.
12. Redline S, Yenokyan G, Gottlieb DJ, et al. Obstructive sleep apnea-hypopnea and incident stroke: the Sleep Heart Health Study. Am J Respir Crit Care Med 2010;182(2):269–77.
13. Hunt NJ, Rodriguez ML, Waters KA, et al. Changes in orexin (hypocretin) neuronal expression with normal aging in the human hypothalamus. Neurobiol Aging 2015;36(1):292–300.
14. Saper CB, Scammell TE, Lu J. Hypothalamic regulation of sleep and circadian rhythms. Nature 2005;437(7063):1257–63.
15. Irwin MR. Sleep and inflammation in resilient aging. Interface Focus 2014;4(5): 20140009.
16. Dean GE, Klimpt ML, Morris JL, et al. Excessive sleepiness. In: Boltz M, Capezuti E, Fulmer T, et al, editors. Evidence-based geriatric nursing protocols for best practice. 5th edition. New York: Springer Publishing Company; 2016. p. 431–42.
17. Schmidt C, Peigneux P, Cajochen C. Age-related changes in sleep and circadian rhythms: impact on cognitive performance and underlying neuroanatomical networks. Front Neurol 2012;3:118.
18. Mattis J, Sehgal A. Circadian rhythms, sleep, and disorders of aging. Trends Endocrinol Metab 2016;27(4):192–203.
19. Rea MS, Figueiro MG, Bierman A, et al. Modelling the spectral sensitivity of the human circadian system. Lighting Res Technology 2012;44(4):386–96.
20. Cajochen C, Munch M, Knoblauch V, et al. Age-related changes in the circadian and homeostatic regulation of human sleep. Chronobiol Int 2006;23(1–2): 461–74.
21. Anderson KN, Catt M, Collerton J, et al. Assessment of sleep and circadian rhythm disorders in the very old: the Newcastle 85+ Cohort Study. Age Ageing 2014;43(1):57–63.
22. Zee PC, Attarian H, Videnovic A. Circadian rhythm abnormalities. Continuum (Minneap Minn) 2013;19(1 Sleep Disorders):132–47.
23. Gooneratne NS, Vitiello MV. Sleep in older adults: normative changes, sleep disorders, and treatment options. Clin Geriatr Med 2014;30(3):591–627.
24. American Psychiatric Association. Diagnostic and statistical manual of mental disorders. 5th edition. Arlington (TX): American Psychiatric Association; 2013.
25. Spielman AJ, Caruso LS, Glovinsky PB. A behavioral perspective on insomnia treatment. Psychiatr Clin North Am 1987;10(4):541–53.

26. Evans DS, Parimi N, Nievergelt CM, et al. Common genetic variants in ARNTL and NPAS2 and at chromosome 12p13 are associated with objectively measured sleep traits in the elderly. Sleep 2013;36(3):431–46.
27. Lovato N, Lack L, Kennaway DJ. Comparing and contrasting therapeutic effects of cognitive-behavior therapy for older adults suffering from insomnia with short and long objective sleep duration. Sleep Med 2016;22:4–12.
28. Perlis ML, Smith LJ, Lyness JM, et al. Insomnia as a risk factor for onset of depression in the elderly. Behav Sleep Med 2006;4(2):104–13.
29. Schwartz S, McDowell Anderson W, Cole SR, et al. Insomnia and heart disease: a review of epidemiologic studies. J Psychosom Res 1999;47(4):313–33.
30. Sigurdardottir LG, Valdimarsdottir UA, Mucci LA, et al. Sleep disruption among older men and risk of prostate cancer. Cancer Epidemiol Biomarkers Prev 2013; 22(5):872–9.
31. Lim AS, Kowgier M, Yu L, et al. Sleep fragmentation and the risk of incident Alzheimer's disease and cognitive decline in older persons. Sleep 2013;36(7): 1027–32.
32. Xiang YT, Weng YZ, Leung CM, et al. Prevalence and correlates of insomnia and its impact on quality of life in Chinese schizophrenia patients. Sleep 2009;32(1): 105–9.
33. Buysse DJ, Germain A, Moul DE, et al. Efficacy of brief behavioral treatment for chronic insomnia in older adults. Arch Intern Med 2011;171(10):887–95.
34. Morin CM, Benca R. Chronic insomnia. Lancet 2012;379(9821):1129–41.
35. American Academy of Sleep Medicine. International classification of sleep disorders, revised: diagnostic and coding manual. 2nd edition. Rochester (MN): American Academy of Sleep Medicine; 2005.
36. Young T, Palta M, Dempsey J, et al. The occurrence of sleep-disordered breathing among middle-aged adults. N Engl J Med 1993;328(17):1230–5.
37. Glasser M, Bailey N, McMillian A, et al. Sleep apnoea in older people. Breathe 2011;7(3):249–56.
38. Tishler PV, Larkin EK, Schluchter MD, et al. Incidence of sleep-disordered breathing in an urban adult population: the relative importance of risk factors in the development of sleep-disordered breathing. JAMA 2003;289(17):2230–7.
39. Eikermann M, Jordan AS, Chamberlin NL, et al. The influence of aging on pharyngeal collapsibility during sleep. Chest 2007;131(6):1702–9.
40. Worsnop C, Kay A, Kim Y, et al. Effect of age on sleep onset-related changes in respiratory pump and upper airway muscle function. J Appl Physiol (1985) 2000;88(5):1831–9.
41. Vazir A, Hastings PC, Dayer M, et al. A high prevalence of sleep disordered breathing in men with mild symptomatic chronic heart failure due to left ventricular systolic dysfunction. Eur J Heart Fail 2007;9(3):243–50.
42. Luyster FS, Choi J, Yeh CH, et al. Screening and evaluation tools for sleep disorders in older adults. Appl Nurs Res 2015;28(4):334–40.
43. Milligan SA, Chesson AL. Restless legs syndrome in the older adult: diagnosis and management. Drugs Aging 2002;19(10):741–51.
44. Allen RP, Picchietti DL, Garcia-Borreguero D, et al. Restless legs syndrome/ Willis-Ekbom disease diagnostic criteria: updated International Restless Legs Syndrome Study Group (IRLSSG) consensus criteria–history, rationale, description, and significance. Sleep Med 2014;15(8):860–73.
45. Boeve BF. REM sleep behavior disorder: Updated review of the core features, the REM sleep behavior disorder-neurodegenerative disease association,

evolving concepts, controversies, and future directions. Ann N Y Acad Sci 2010; 1184:15–54.

46. Ohayon MM, Caulet M, Priest RG. Violent behavior during sleep. J Clin Psychiatry 1997;58(8):369–76 [quiz: 377].

47. Vaz Fragoso CA, Gahbauer EA, Van Ness PH, et al. Sleep-wake disturbances and frailty in community-living older persons. J Am Geriatr Soc 2009;57(11): 2094–100.

48. Zhu L, Zee PC. Circadian rhythm sleep disorders. Neurol Clin 2012;30(4): 1167–91.

49. Barion A, Zee PC. A clinical approach to circadian rhythm sleep disorders. Sleep Med 2007;8(6):566–77.

50. Buysse DJ. Insomnia state of the science: an evolutionary, evidence-based assessment. Sleep 2005;28(9):1045–6.

51. Bain KT. Management of chronic insomnia in elderly persons. Am J Geriatr Pharmacother 2006;4(2):168–92.

52. Schroeck JL, Ford J, Conway EL, et al. Review of safety and efficacy of sleep medicines in older adults. Clin Ther 2016;38(11):2340–72.

53. Culpepper L. Secondary insomnia in the primary care setting: review of diagnosis, treatment, and management. Curr Med Res Opin 2006;22(7):1257–68.

54. American Geriatrics Society 2015 Beers Criteria Update Expert Panel. American Geriatrics Society 2015 updated Beers criteria for potentially inappropriate medication use in older adults. J Am Geriatr Soc 2015;63(11):2227–46.

55. Somers VK, White DP, Amin R, et al. Sleep Apnea and Cardiovascular Disease. An American Heart Association/American College of Cardiology Foundation Scientific Statement from the American Heart Association Council for High Blood Pressure Research Professional Education Committee, Council on Clinical Cardiology, Stroke Council, and Council on Cardiovascular Nursing Council. Circulation 2008;118:1080–111.

56. Stone KL, Blackwell TL, Ancoli-Israel S, et al. Sleep disordered breathing and risk of stroke in older community-dwelling men. Sleep 2016;39(3):531–40.

57. Bradley TD, Floras JS. Obstructive sleep apnoea and its cardiovascular consequences. Lancet 2009;373(9657):82–93.

58. Das AM, Khayat R. Hypertension in obstructive sleep apnea: risk and therapy. Expert Rev Cardiovasc Ther 2009;7(6):619–26.

59. Luthje L, Andreas S. Obstructive sleep apnea and coronary artery disease. Sleep Med Rev 2008;12(1):19–31.

60. Prinz C, Bitter T, Piper C, et al. Sleep apnea is common in patients with coronary artery disease. Wien Med Wochenschr 2010;160(13–14):349–55.

61. Shah NA, Yaggi HK, Concato J, et al. Obstructive sleep apnea as a risk factor for coronary events or cardiovascular death. Sleep Breath 2010;14(2):131–6.

62. Tamura A, Kawano Y, Ando S, et al. Association between coronary spastic angina pectoris and obstructive sleep apnea. J Cardiol 2010;56(2):240–4.

63. Skomro RP, Ludwig S, Salamon E, et al. Sleep complaints and restless legs syndrome in adult type 2 diabetics. Sleep Med 2001;2(5):417–22.

64. Foster GD, Sanders MH, Millman R, et al. Obstructive sleep apnea among obese patients with type 2 diabetes. Diabetes Care 2009;32(6):1017–9.

65. Lam DC, Lui MM, Lam JC, et al. Prevalence and recognition of obstructive sleep apnea in Chinese patients with type 2 diabetes mellitus. Chest 2010;138(5): 1101–7.

66. Budhiraja R, Roth T, Hudgel DW, et al. Prevalence and polysomnographic correlates of insomnia comorbid with medical disorders. Sleep 2011;34(7):859–67.

67. Dahiya S, Ahluwalia MS, Walia HK. Sleep disturbances in cancer patients: underrecognized and undertreated. Cleveland Clinic J Med 2013;80(11): 722–32.
68. Morin CM, LeBlanc M, Belanger L, et al. Prevalence of insomnia and its treatment in Canada. Can J Psychiatry 2011;56(9):540–8.
69. Savard J, Morin CM. Insomnia in the context of cancer: a review of a neglected problem. J Clin Oncol 2001;19(3):895–908.
70. Omachi TA, Blanc PD, Claman DM, et al. Disturbed sleep among COPD patients is longitudinally associated with mortality and adverse COPD outcomes. Sleep Med 2012;13(5):476–83.
71. Son CN, Choi G, Lee SY, et al. Sleep quality in rheumatoid arthritis, and its association with disease activity in a Korean population. Korean J Intern Med 2015;30(3):384–90.
72. Smagula SF, Boudreau RM, Stone K, et al. Latent activity rhythm disturbance sub-groups and longitudinal change in depression symptoms among older men. Chronobiol Int 2015;32(10):1427–37.
73. Wang JL, Lim AS, Chiang W-Y, et al. Suprachiasmatic neuron numbers and rest-activity circadian rhythms in older humans. Ann Neurol 2015;78(2):317–22.
74. Kondratova AA, Kondratov RV. The circadian clock and pathology of the ageing brain. Nat Rev Neurosci 2012;13(5):325–35.
75. Leblanc MF, Desjardins S, Desgagne A. Sleep problems in anxious and depressive older adults. Psychol Res Behav Manag 2015;8:161–9.
76. Becker NB, Jesus SN, Joao KA, et al. Depression and sleep quality in older adults: a meta-analysis. Psychol Health Med 2016. [Epub ahead or print].
77. Larsson C, Hansson EE, Sundquist K, et al. Chronic pain in older adults: prevalence, incidence, and risk factors. Scand J Rheumatol 2016. [Epub ahead or print].
78. Vitiello MV, Rybarczyk B, Von Korff M, et al. Cognitive behavioral therapy for insomnia improves sleep and decreases pain in older adults with co-morbid insomnia and osteoarthritis. J Clin Sleep Med 2009;5(4):355–62.
79. Finan PH, Goodin BR, Smith MT. The association of sleep and pain: an update and a path forward. J Pain 2013;14(12):1539–52.
80. Chen Q, Hayman LL, Shmerling RH, et al. Characteristics of chronic pain associated with sleep difficulty in older adults: the Maintenance of Balance, Independent Living, Intellect, and Zest in the Elderly (MOBILIZE) Boston study. J Am Geriatr Soc 2011;59(8):1385–92.
81. Taylor DJ, Mallory LJ, Lichstein KL, et al. Comorbidity of chronic insomnia with medical problems. Sleep 2007;30(2):213–8.
82. Bosch JL, Weiss JP. The prevalence and causes of nocturia. J Urol 2013;189(1 Suppl):S86–92.
83. Madhu C, Coyne K, Hashim H, et al. Nocturia: risk factors and associated comorbidities; findings from the EpiLUTS study. Int J Clin Pract 2015;69(12): 1508–16.
84. Chasens ER, Umlauf MG. Nocturia: a problem that disrupts sleep and predicts obstructive sleep apnea. Geriatr Nurs 2003;24(2):76–81, 105.
85. Morris JL, Sereika SM, Houze M, et al. Effect of nocturia on next-day sedentary activity in adults with type 2 diabetes. Appl Nurs Res 2016;32:44–6.
86. Rafiq M, McGovern A, Jones S, et al. Falls in the elderly were predicted opportunistically using a decision tree and systematically using a database-driven screening tool. J Clin Epidemiol 2014;67(8):877–86.

87. Pallesen S, Sivertsen B, Nordhus IH, et al. A 10-year trend of insomnia prevalence in the adult Norwegian population. Sleep Med 2014;15(2):173–9.
88. Fonareva I, Oken BS. Physiological and functional consequences of caregiving for relatives with dementia. Int Psychogeriatr 2014;26(5):725–47.
89. Jain FA, Nazarian N, Lavretsky H. Feasibility of central meditation and imagery therapy for dementia caregivers. Int J Geriatr Psychiatry 2014;29(8):870–6.
90. Paller KA, Creery JD, Florczak SM, et al. Benefits of mindfulness training for patients with progressive cognitive decline and their caregivers. Am J Alzheimers Dis Other Demen 2015;30(3):257–67.
91. Arber S, Bote M, Meadows R. Gender and socio-economic patterning of self-reported sleep problems in Britain. Soc Sci Med 2009;68(2):281–9.
92. Troxel WM, Robles TF, Hall M, et al. Marital quality and the marital bed: examining the covariation between relationship quality and sleep. Sleep Med Rev 2007;11(5):389–404.
93. van de Straat V, Bracke P. How well does Europe sleep? A cross-national study of sleep problems in European older adults. Int J Public Health 2015;60(6): 643–50.
94. Knauert MP, Malik V, Kamdar BB. Sleep and sleep disordered breathing in hospitalized patients. Semin Respir Crit Care Med 2014;35(5):582–92.
95. Missildine K, Bergstrom N, Meininger J, et al. Sleep in hospitalized elders: a pilot study. Geriatr Nurs 2010;31(4):263–71.
96. Spence J, Murray T, Tang AS, et al. Nighttime noise issues that interrupt sleep after cardiac surgery. J Nurs Care Qual 2011;26(1):88–95.
97. Freedman NS, Gazendam J, Levan L, et al. Abnormal sleep/wake cycles and the effect of environmental noise on sleep disruption in the intensive care unit. Am J Respir Crit Care Med 2001;163(2):451–7.
98. Figueroa-Ramos MI, Arroyo-Novoa CM, Lee KA, et al. Sleep and delirium in ICU patients: a review of mechanisms and manifestations. Intensive Care Med 2009; 35(5):781–95.
99. Kamdar BB, Needham DM, Collop NA. Sleep deprivation in critical illness: its role in physical and psychological recovery. J Intensive Care Med 2012;27(2): 97–111.
100. Edinger JD, Carney CE. Overcoming insomnia: a cognitive-behavioral therapy approach—therapist guide. (Treatments that Work). New York: Oxford University Press; 2015.
101. Garfield V, Llewellyn CH, Kumari M. The relationship between physical activity, sleep duration and depressive symptoms in older adults: the English Longitudinal Study of Ageing (ELSA). Prev Med Rep 2016;4:512–6.
102. Bankar MA, Chaudhari SK, Chaudhari KD. Impact of long term yoga practice on sleep quality and quality of life in the elderly. J Ayurveda Integr Med 2013;4(1): 28–32.
103. Du S, Dong J, Zhang H, et al. Taichi exercise for self-rated sleep quality in older people: a systematic review and meta-analysis. Int J Nurs Stud 2015;52(1): 368–79.
104. Campos Costa I, Nogueira Carvalho H, Fernandes L. Aging, circadian rhythms and depressive disorders: a review. Am J Neurodegener Dis 2013;2(4):228–46.
105. Kuramoto AM. Therapeutic benefits of Tai Chi exercise: research review. WMJ 2006;105(7):42–6.
106. Fanning J, Porter G, Awick EA, et al. Replacing sedentary time with sleep, light, or moderate-to-vigorous physical activity: effects on self-regulation and executive functioning. J Behav Med 2016;40(2):332–42.

107. Endeshaw YW, Yoo W. Association between social and physical activities and insomnia symptoms among community-dwelling older adults. J Aging Health 2016;28(6):1073–89.
108. Dimsdale JE, Norman D, DeJardin D, et al. The effect of opioids on sleep architecture. J Clin Sleep Med 2007;3(1):33–6.
109. Lenz TL. Drugs that negatively affect sleep. Am J Lifestyle Med 2014;8(6): 383–5.
110. Ozdemir PG, Karadag AS, Selvi Y, et al. Assessment of the effects of antihistamine drugs on mood, sleep quality, sleepiness, and dream anxiety. Int J Psychiatry Clin Pract 2014;18(3):161–8.
111. Shah C, Sharma TR, Kablinger A. Controversies in the use of second generation antipsychotics as sleep agent. Pharmacol Res 2014;79:1–8.

Impairments in Skin Integrity

Rose W. Murphree, DNP, MSN, RN, CWOCN, CFCN

KEYWORDS

- Skin integrity • Wounds • Pressure ulcer or injury • Skin tears • Ulcers

KEY POINTS

- Maintenance of skin integrity during the elder years is a challenge for most people. Maintaining skin in a supple and moist condition can help prevent many skin injuries.
- Intrinsic factors, such as altered nutrition, vascular disease issues, and diabetes, can affect skin integrity. Limiting risk factors throughout the lifespan will help reduce likelihood of impaired skin integrity.
- Extrinsic factors, such as falls and other accidents, pressure, and surgical procedures, also affect skin integrity. Addressing these factors requires efforts from the individual, family, and clinicians.
- Many evidence-based tools now available online assist clinicians with determining appropriate treatment plans when altered skin integrity exists.

INTRODUCTION

A discussion of impairments in skin integrity can only begin with an overview of the integumentary system. Often, integumentary and skin are used interchangeably; however, there is a distinct difference between them. The integumentary system has 3 distinct layers: epidermis, dermis, and hypodermis or subcutaneous.[1,2] Covering approximately 21 square feet, skin (or integument) is the largest organ of the integumentary system and combines the epidermis and dermis layers.[1,2]

Skin critically functions to maintain homeostasis of our internal environment while also protecting us from the external environment. In its optimal state, skin is soft, dry, supple, and intact. It is acidic in nature with a pH between 4 and 6.8. On a cellular level, skin configuration is similar to brick and mortar, with the skin cells resembling bricks and skin lipids (oils) resembling mortar. Ceramide is the most abundant type of skin lipid and helps create the barrier functionality of skin. Keratinocytes produce skin lipids and help maintain skin hydration, filling in the gaps between the skin cells creating intact skin.[1,2]

Properly hydrated skin cells maintain normal contours. Conversely, dry skin cells have a shrunken appearance, whereas overhydrated cells are edematous or swollen.

Disclosure Statement: The author has nothing to disclose.
Wound, Ostomy, and Continence Nursing Education Center, Emory University, Nell Hodgson Woodruff School of Nursing, 1520 Clifton Road NE, Atlanta, GA 30322, USA
E-mail address: Rose.Murphree@emory.edu

Any abnormal hydration compromises the barrier effect and tensile strength is compromised with overhydration. Transepidermal water loss (TEWL) is an indicator of the skin's barrier function and integrity.[1] An increase in the TEWL value is indicator of compromised skin.[1,2] Appropriate skin care products should be able to keep the skin dry, supple, and acidic.

Clinicians receive a good overview, albeit brief, of the integumentary system during their undergraduate education. Only those clinicians who choose to specialize in wound care, ostomy care, and/or continence care delve into the integumentary system beyond skin. The purpose of this article is to provide the clinician with a deeper understanding of skin, the integumentary system, and current concepts for maintaining intact skin in hopes of promoting positive patient outcomes, regardless of the health care delivery setting. This article explores the extrinsic and intrinsic factors that can lead to impairment of skin integrity and introduces the clinician to current treatment strategies. A brief overview of dressing options for each impairment of skin integrity issue is explained; however, in-depth discussion of wound healing principles and wound dressings is beyond the scope of this article.

ANATOMY AND PHYSIOLOGY OF A HEALTHY INTEGUMENTARY SYSTEM

The outermost layer of skin is the epidermis. This layer provides protection from the external environment. It is approximately 20 cells thick with 4 and 5 sublayers.[1] The stratified squamous epithelial cells, or keratinocytes, range in thickness from 75 to 150 μm (0.4–0.6 mm on the soles of the feet and palms of the hands).[1,2] **Table 1** provides a brief description of these sublayers.

Table 1
Sublayers of the epidermis

Sublayer	Alternative Name	Description	Function
Stratum corneum	Horny layer	• Outermost layer • Composed of dead keratinocytes filled with protein keratin • Constantly sloughed off and replenished by sublayers beneath	Barrier against penetration by irritants or pathogens
Stratum lucidum	—	• Only present on soles of feet and palms of hands	Provides thickness on soles of feet and palms of hands
Stratum granulosum	—	• 1–5 cells thick • Ceramides from Odland bodies (found in keratinocytes) are released from this layer	Ceramides form a lipophilic layer that maintains hydrations and slows water loss
Stratum spinosum	Prickly layer	• Contains desmosomes or cell to cell junctions	Provides cellular adhesion and resistance to mechanical forces
Stratum germinativum	Stratum basale	• Single layer of reproducing cells • Basal cell division results in 2 cells: keratinocytes and another reproducing basal cell	Keratinocytes migrate toward the stratum corneum and become filled with keratin

The epidermis contains cells that add skin pigmentation and aid the immune system. Capillary loops from the dermis layer provide nutrients and oxygenation to the epidermal cells. Nerve receptors extend to the epidermis and provide tactile sensations of pain, pressure, touch, temperature, and so forth.[1,2] **Table 2** provides an overview of these cells and receptors.

The epidermis and dermis layers are connected through an intricate interlocking system whereby the rete ridges of the epidermal layer project downward, whereas the dermal papillae project upward. This area is commonly called the basement membrane zone or dermal-epidermal junction. This cohesive mechanism provides a unified movement of the 2 layers. Disruption of the dermal-epidermal junction occurs with blister formation.[1,2]

The dermis layer, sometimes referred to as corium, has 2 sublayers: papillary dermis, which provides capillary loops to the epidermis; and reticular dermis, which contains an extensive vascular plexus, lymphatics, and connective tissue proteins. The epidermal appendages, such as hair follicles, sweat glands, nerves, and sebaceous glands, are located in the reticular dermis area. Epidermal appendages are lined with epidermis. This is significant in wound healing because intact epidermal membrane in the appendages results in re-epithelialization without scarring and is often noted as partial-thickness tissue loss. Key cells necessary for wound healing processes are located throughout the dermis layer.[1,2] **Table 3** provides an overview of the sublayers, key cells, and epidermal appendages.

The deepest layer of the integumentary system is the hypodermis, more commonly called subcutaneous or adipose tissue. Hypodermis contains adipose and connective tissues, blood and lymphatic vessels, and nerve endings. This layer provides cushioning against pressure and shear forces. Tissue destruction to this level, known as full-thickness tissue loss, results in granulation tissue development to fill the defect and scar formation because subcutaneous tissue cannot be regenerated.[1,2]

Table 2		
Other components within the epidermis layer		
Component	**Function**	**Interesting Factoid**
Melanocytes	Provide skin pigmentation Provide protection from harmful ultraviolet rays	Light- and dark-skinned people have approximately same number of melanocytes Melanin pigment produces variation in color
Nerve receptors	Provide sensitivity to temperature, touch, pressure, pain	Merkel cells are named for Friedrich Sigmund Merkel who identified them as touch cells Largest number found on fingertips
Rete ridges	Form the dermal-epidermal junction to provide contiguous movement of dermis and epidermis layers	Convoluted borders of epidermis project downward and interlock with upward projecting dermal papillae
Blood vessels	Nonexistent	Nutrient and oxygenation of epidermal cells occurs from capillary loops found within the papillary dermis
Langerhans cells	Provide antigens that help the skin immune system	Most prominent in the stratum spinosum, but present in all layers of epidermis except stratum corneum Also found in papillary dermis

Table 3
Components of dermis

Component	Subcomponents	Function or Description
Dermal layers	Papillary dermis	Dermal papillae interlock with rete ridges Dermal papillae contain capillary loops responsible for nutrient delivery and oxygenation of stratum germinativum layer of epidermis
	Reticular dermis	Beneath papillary dermis Provides vascular plexus, lymphatics, and connective tissue proteins like collagen
Key cells	Fibroblasts	Synthesize connective tissue proteins (elastin and collagen) Collagen provides tensile strength to skin, whereas elastin provides recoil or memory (stretch)
	Macrophages	Phagocytic cells derived from monocytes Provide defense against pathogens
	Mast cells	Produce histamine and other proteins Results in inflammation
Nerve cells	Receptors terminate in epidermis	Provide sensation for pain, touch, pressure, and temperature
Epidermal appendages	Hair follicles	Hair growth occurs from root Tissue destruction below root area results in no hair Contain arrectores pilorum (tiny muscles) that cause goose bumps when stimulated
	Sebaceous glands	Produce sebum (lipids and triglycerides) that lubricates and waterproofs the skin
	Sweat glands	Secrete sweat that helps regulate body temperature

Data from Emory University Wound, Ostomy, and Continence Nursing Education Center's wound core curriculum. Atlanta (GA): Emory University WOCNEC; 2016. p. 1–312; and Mufti A, Ayello EA, Sibbald RG. Anatomy and physiology of the skin. In: Doughty DB, McNichol LL, editors. Wound, Ostomy, and Continence Nurses Society core curriculum: wound management. Philadelphia: Wolters Kluwer; 2016. p. 3–23.

An intact and optimum integumentary system provides protection against pathogens, irritants, and fluid loss; as well as temperature regulation through vasoconstriction and shivering, and vasodilation and sweating. Excretion of hypotonic fluid, sweat, can range from 100 mL in 1 day to 2 L in 1 hour. Sensory perception, information and protection, arises through the complex nerve receptors. Exposure to sunlight aids in vitamin D synthesis.[1,2] Although not tangible, the integumentary system serves as a form of expression and body image.

Normal epidermis contains resident bacteria. Overgrowth or undergrowth of these bacteria can occur with excess moisture, antibiotic regimen, alkaline soaps, and dysfunction of the immune system. Transient bacteria, which are normally not found on the skin, are generally removed by routine cleansing. Improper wound cultures can result in contaminated results and lead to inappropriate treatment plans; therefore, adequate flushing of a wound bed is required before swabbing for a culture. A wound culture is recommended when erythema and induration persist more than 2 cm from the wound edge, and the culture should be obtained from viable wound bed tissue, not the drainage in the wound, when a dressing is removed.[1]

Keratinocytes of the epidermis slough daily at a rate of about 0.024 to 0.072 ounces.[3] Even with this amount of cell loss each day, normal turnover of skin cells takes about 20 days. In the elderly population, the turnover rate is prolonged to about 30 days.[1] As a result of this delayed epidermal mitosis in the elderly, the epidermal skin layers are much thinner than a healthy child.

CHANGES IN INTEGUMENTARY SYSTEM DUE TO AGING

The changes in the integumentary system as one ages places the individual at higher risk for infectious processes, tissue destruction, and other disease processes. These changes also increase risks for extrinsic factors to result in tissue destruction. Increased awareness of these normal changes can assist the clinician to monitor the elderly skin and risk factors more closely.

A decreased barrier function increases the risk of penetration by pathogens, and irritation occurs with epidermal thinning and drier skin, which is due to reduced activity of sebaceous and sweat glands. Rete ridges and dermal papillae flatten, which causes decreased cohesion of the dermal-epidermal junction and increases risk of skin tears.[1,2] Collagen bundles shrink, causing wrinkles. Gray hair and senile lentigo (age spots) are the results of erratic or decreased melanin production. Decrease thermal insulation and increased risk for shear and pressure injuries occur because subcutaneous tissue is thinner.[1,2] The elderly are also at higher risk for injury due to decreased sensory receptors.

Other integumentary issues for elderly include

1. Delayed wound healing because there is a reduction in blood flow and increased time for epidermal cell turnover
2. Impaired capillary fragility that increases occurrence of purpura or bruising
3. Increased incidence in premalignant and malignant lesions
4. Increased cell senescence or decreased cell competence, causing an inability for cells to reproduce or provide essential repair activities
5. Increased expression of inflammatory mediators and decreased expression of inflammatory inhibitors, resulting in delayed wound healing.

Clinicians and caregivers for the elderly can address these normal alterations of the integumentary system with a comprehensive skin health plan. Strategies such as individualized plans for bathing frequency, pH-balanced soaps for skin types, and applying moisturizing products while skin is still damp can help improve and maintain skin integrity for the elderly.[4] **Table 4** notes a few products considerations for routine cleansing

Table 4	
Products to promote skin health in the elderly	
Focus	**Products**
Skin cleansing	pH-balanced cleansers
	pH-balanced no-rinse impregnated in soft disposable cloths
	Superfatted nonalkaline soaps for individuals with dry skin
	Disposable bathing systems impregnated with chlorhexidine gluconate for high-risk patient populations
Skin moisturization	Emollients: increase lipid component, add softness, delay water loss on skin surface, help keep stratum corneum cells plump
	Examples: mineral oil, petrolatum, lanolin, ceramides, dimethicone, vegetable oil (Schleicher, 2015)[4]
	Humectants: pull water into the epidermal cells, increase water component of the stratum corneum; best for individuals with very dry skin or xerosis; contraindicated for macerated skin and fragile skin
	Examples: glycerin, urea, propylene glycol, Lac-Hydrin, alpha hydroxy acids

Data from Emory University Wound, Ostomy, and Continence Nursing Education Center's wound core curriculum. Atlanta (GA): Emory University WOCNEC; 2016. p. 11; and Mufti A, Ayello EA, Sibbald RG. Anatomy and physiology of the skin. In: Doughty DB, McNichol LL, editors. Wound, Ostomy, and Continence Nurses Society core curriculum: wound management. Philadelphia: Wolters Kluwer; 2016. p. 19.

and moisturization of the skin. Occasionally, skin problems arise that are beyond routine skin cleansing care. Although **Table 5** offers some management options for these problematic skin issues, clinicians should refer individuals to dermatology specialists when these strategies are ineffective or prescription formulas are needed.[1,2,4]

IMPAIRMENTS IN SKIN INTEGRITY

Although impairments in skin integrity can occur along the age continuum, elderly individuals are particularly vulnerable by virtue of the changes previously noted. Most clinicians equate the nursing diagnosis of impairment in skin integrity to pressure ulcers or injuries, but it can also be several other factors. Regardless of the impairment, effective treatment principles are a must for every clinician. The first step is to identify the etiologic factors, or what specifically is causing the impairment. This requires a thorough assessment of the individual, not just the impairment. The comprehensive assessment should include medical history, current medical status, medications, and identification of any family medical issues. The comprehensive assessment helps to identify specific risk factors, as well as identify potential systemic issues that may delay wound healing. Addressing both the etiologic factors and systemic factors, in addition to appropriate topical therapy, will aid the clinician in a more successful wound management approach. Impairment in skin integrity issues require a comprehensive team approach, and referrals to certified wound care clinicians will enhance this team approach and assure appropriate wound healing principles are initiated for optimum treatment.[5]

IMPAIRMENTS IN SKIN INTEGRITY COMMONLY SEEN IN ELDERLY
Friction Rubs, Abrasions, and Blisters

Friction rubs, abrasions, and blisters are a result of repetitive friction during movement in a bed or chair, or excessive scrubbing of the skin. The resultant loss of the top few

Table 5
Problematic skin management

Problem	Management Strategies
Pruritic (itchy) skin	Reduce bathing frequency Use tepid water for bathing Use soothing products for bath soaks Examples: AVEENO Soothing Bath Treatment (oatmeal base); Burow's Solution (aluminum triacetate) Apply emollients after bathing
Dry, scaly skin (particularly diabetic feet)	Soak in vinegar and water solution (1 part vinegar to 3 parts water) Lightly buff skin after soaking Apply emollients and humectants in combination after bathing Examples: urea-based products (Lac-Hydrin, Atrac-Tain), modified petrolatum products (Elta, Aquaphor)
Thin fragile skin	Use soft cloths and gentle care for bathing Moisturize after bathing Limit adhesive products on skin Use protective wraps on elbows, knees

Data from Emory University Wound, Ostomy, and Continence Nursing Education Center's wound core curriculum. Atlanta (GA): Emory University WOCNEC; 2016. p. 1–312; and Mufti A, Ayello EA, Sibbald RG. Anatomy and physiology of the skin. In: Doughty DB, McNichol LL, editors. Wound, Ostomy, and Continence Nurses Society core curriculum: wound management. Philadelphia: Wolters Kluwer; 2016. p. 3–23.

sublayers of epidermal cells initiates an inflammatory response of the remaining sublayers and is evidenced by erythema and tenderness of intact skin. This response may precede actual tissue loss that results in dermis exposure. It is a very common response in the presence of macerated or fragile skin.

A thorough assessment of the individual's activity status may reveal use of restraints, frequent motion against rough linens or chair cloths, use of adult briefs for incontinence issues, or repetitive rubbing of limbs, especially when heel blisters occur. Recurrent friction injury in the sacral areas may result in superficial skin loss and simultaneous thickening of skin the area (or lichenification).

Using soft bathing cloths, gentle skin care, heel elevation devices (even while in a recliner), and support surface and/or linens with low friction and low shear coverings will help prevent friction rubs from occurring. Applying protective dressings, such as protective sleeves to elbows, transparent adhesive dressings to heels or elbows, and/or silicone adhesive foam dressings to the sacrococcygeal area will also encourage intact skin. Open lesions due to friction tend to be partial-thickness and usually have minimal exudate. Dressing management goals focus to absorb exudate, keep the wound surface moist, and prevent further trauma. Specific dressing suggestions are noted in **Table 6** in the section for partial-thickness and dry wounds.

Skin Tears

A recent systematic review[5] found skin tears most frequently occur among individuals who are elderly, depend on others for care, and with limited mobility. The prevalence ranged between 3.3% and 22% in acute care settings, whereas prevalence in home care ranged between 5.5% and 19.5%.[6] The disruption between skin layers, primarily the epidermis and dermis, occurs when the layers slide against each other. Thinned skin and flattened rete ridges decrease the dermal-epidermal junction.[1,2]

The International Skin Tear Advisory Panel (ISTAP)[7] has created a classification for skin tears based on amount of tissue loss. No skin loss is associated with a type 1 skin tear. The edges of the flap can be approximated and the flap is viable, so

Table 6
Dressings based on wound characteristics

Wound Characteristics	Dressing Options
Partial-thickness or shallow wound with minimal amount of drainage	Hydrocolloid, thin or regular thickness Oil-emersion with gauze covering Silicone-type dressing Nonadherent adhesive bandage Transparent adhesive dressing Wound gel to add moisture
Partial-thickness or shallow wound with large amount of drainage	Alginate or hydrofiber with cover dressing Silicone-type foam
Full-thickness or deep wound with large amount of dressing	Alginate or hydrofiber with cover dressing Foam dressing Nonwoven gauze with cover dressing
Full-thickness or deep wound with minimal amount of drainage	Alginate or hydrofiber covered by transparent adhesive dressing Wound gel with moistened gauze dressing and cover dressing

Modified from Emory University Wound, Ostomy, and Continence Nursing Education Center's wound core curriculum. Atlanta (GA): Emory University WOCNEC; 2016. p. 1–312; with permission.

uncomplicated healing is anticipated. A type 2 skin tear only has a partial skin flap present. A type 3 skin tear has total loss of skin and/or no viable flap. ISTAP offers a Skin Tear Toolkit and decision algorithm for clinicians (http://www.skintears.org/Skin-Tear-Tool-Kit/).[8] Dressing management of skin tear wounds is very similar to friction wounds. Primary concerns for clinicians are prevention of more skin tears and protection of any viable flaps in the skin tear wound. The best options for skin tear dressings include a nonadherent emulsion gauze or silicone-type dressing with a light-weight pad and gauze wrap. Gentle care and skin handling is a must. Prevention of trauma by padding bedrails and wheelchairs is also helpful. Given that some skin tears are caused by tape removal, see later discussion for more information about medical adhesive–related skin injury (MARSI).[1,2,7]

Medical Adhesive–Related Skin Injuries

MARSIs are defined as erythema and/or other indicators of skin damage (eg, blisters, skin tears, and folliculitis) that persists for 30 minutes after removal of an adhesive product.[9] Products causing MARSI include tape, adhesive dressings, ostomy appliances with adhesive backing, and so forth. Frail, elderly, and individuals with thin fragile skin due to drugs, malnutrition, or dermatologic conditions, and/or on cytotoxic therapies (radiation or chemotherapies) are among the highest risk population.[9] Critical care, emergency, and operating room areas also have increased risk for creating MARSIs. The primary mechanism of injury is mechanical trauma or stripping, but contact dermatitis and maceration can also cause MARSI.[1,2,9]

Prevention is the primary management focus. Decreasing the use of aggressive adhesive products is a must. Assuring correct removal technique is also helpful. This is done as a low and slow technique, supporting the skin adjacent to the adhesive product and avoiding rapid removal.[9] When possible, use of nonadherent products is encouraged.[9] Open lesions tend to be partial-thickness wounds and treatment follows the shallow-dry wound section of **Table 6**.

Moisture-Associated Skin Damage

There are 4 types of moisture-associated skin damage (MASD): incontinence-associated dermatitis (IAD), intertriginous dermatitis (ITD), periwound MASD, and peristomal MASD. Prolonged or repetitive exposure to moisture (eg, stool, urine, wound drainage, and perspiration) is a contributing factor to MASD.[1,2] The source of moisture is internal for ITD, whereas the other MASD issues have external moisture. All types begin with inflammatory changes of erythema and tenderness, with progression to skin loss with prolonged exposure. Often, the normal bacterial flora is imbalanced to the point that an underlying fungal rash develops.[1,2]

Prevention and management are primarily focused on eliminating exposure of skin to the moisture. IAD is best treated with application of moisture barrier products, including petrolatum-based ointments, dimethicone-based creams, zinc oxide-based ointments, or a combination of products.[1,2] One study of nursing home patients examined the application of an alcohol-free liquid barrier film 3 times a week for perineal skin care.[5] The results found a decrease in IAD occurrence, decreased nursing time for incontinence care, and decreased product utilization.[5]

ITD is a linear break that occurs in the base of skin folds and is caused by overhydration of the skin due to trapped moisture (perspiration) and friction exerted by opposing skin folds.[1,2] This often occurs during cleansing and assessment. Treatment of ITD is focused at wicking or absorbing the excess moisture within the skin folds. Treatment options include placing pads, soft cloths, or pillowcases between the skin folds. The commercial product InterDry (Coloplast US) is available with and without silver to combat any fungal or bacterial infection that could be present.[10]

Both periwound MASD and peristomal MASD are caused by excessive exposure to effluent from the wound, fistula, and/or stoma.[1,2] Treatment of both focuses on disrupting the exposure. Using a dressing that manages the effluent from the wound will help protect periwound skin. Helping clinicians realize dressing changes may need to occur more frequently if the drainage overwhelms the dressing is a priority. Assuring an ostomy pouch addresses the contour challenges in peristomal spaces will help remedy peristomal MASD.[1] Because both dressings and pouching appliances are adhesive-based products, a preliminary application of pectin or antifungal powder, followed by dabbing or blotting a skin sealant atop the powder, will aid in creating a dry surface on which the adhesive product can stick. The dressing and/or pouch may need to be changed more frequently until the skin re-epithelializes. Referrals to a certified wound and/or ostomy clinician will help provide positive outcomes for individuals with MASD issues.

Pressure-Related Injuries

The terms decubitus ulcer, decubiti, bedsore, pressure ulcer, and so forth, are no longer used to describe tissue damage caused by pressure.[1,11] The National Pressure Ulcer Advisory Panel[11] has revised terms with the recommendation of the term injury rather than ulcer. This change has been endorsed by the Wound, Ostomy, and Continence Nurse (WOCN) Society and is reflected in the WOCN guidelines for pressure ulcers or injuries.[12]

Pressure injury is currently considered an area of tissue destruction over a boney prominence within the muscle-bone interface. Muscle is the most metabolically active tissue layer, which makes it the most vulnerable to ischemic injury when intense or prolonged periods of pressure occur. Inactivity due to illness and/or mobility issues, such as arthritis, increases the development of pressure injuries in the elderly population.[11,12]

Prevention is the best management of pressure injuries. Several evidence-based risk assessment tools are available to help clinicians identify those at risk for development of a pressure injury.[11,12] The Braden Pressure Ulcer Risk Assessment Tool[1,13,14] is available online and used in most health care institutions. Helping clinicians use the information gleaned with a risk assessment tool is key to prevention. **Box 1** identifies recognized risk factors used by these assessment tools. Involving all members of the health care team, the individual, and their caregiver is another primary strategy in preventing of pressure injury development.

Individuals identified at risk of pressure injury development or who have healed pressure injury sites will need evaluation for pressure redistributing surfaces to assist with offloading pressure.[15,16] Identifying the correct support surface can be a daunting task. The Support Surface Algorithm (SSA) from WOCN is an evidence-based tool that helps the clinician determine a strong protocol for addressing pressure injuries.[16] The SSA can be accessed using any Internet search engine at http://www. supportsurfacealgorithm.com/www.supportsurfacealgorithm.com.[16]

A strong prevention program[1,15] should include the following:

- Routine assessment using a risk-assessment tool
- Use of pressure redistribution devices: bed and chair
- Schedule and guidelines for repositioning: bed and chair; even with pressure redistribution devices; every 2 hours body shifts in bed and 1 hour in chair if no injuries present

---

Box 1
Recognized risk factors for pressure injury development (listed alphabetically)

Age

Compromised sensation and/or level of consciousness

Exposure to shear and friction

General debility or endstage disease

Hypotension

Incontinence or excessive moisture (eg, sweating, wound drainage)

Increased body temperature

Intractable pain

Malnutrition, especially poor protein intake

Poor perfusion

Prolonged surgical procedure

Restricted activity or mobility

Smoking

Use of vasopressors

From Emory University Wound, Ostomy, and Continence Nursing Education Center's wound core curriculum. Atlanta (GA): Emory University WOCNEC; 2016. p. 1–312.

- Measures for reduction of shear and friction exposure: lift sheets, low friction or shear linens, protective dressings such as soft silicone foam dressings
- Measures to address incontinence or maceration issues
- Routine assessment of and intervention for nutritional status
- Assessment and documentation of skin status at least daily.

Addressing open pressure injuries, as with other wounds, is based on wound size and characteristics. **Table 7** assists the clinician with dressing options to consider with pressure injury management. Referrals to a certified wound care clinician will help identify best practices and options for wound management.[5] Wound management resources include

- *WOCN Guidelines for Prevention and Management of Pressure Ulcers (Injuries)*[12]
- *WOCN Core Curriculum: Wound Management.*[1]

Vascular Impairment

Vascular issues include arterial, venous, and neuropathic issues. Some individuals may present with a combination of these issues. Differential diagnosis requires a thorough assessment of medical, family, pain, wound, and treatment history. Identifying the cause of the wound, evaluating systemic issues that may be delaying wound healing process, and applying appropriate topical therapy are critical to wound healing when vascular issues are present. **Table 8** provides a quick overview of presentation and treatment focus with vascular-related skin impairment.

Other resources available for the clinician to assure appropriate treatment protocols are instituted are

- The WOCN evidence-based and consensus-based algorithm for care across the continuum, *Compression for Primary Prevention, Treatment, and Prevention of*

Table 7
Stages of pressure ulcers or injuries from the National Pressure Ulcer Advisory Panel

Pressure Injury Title	Description
Stage 1	Nonblanchable erythema; dark pigmented skin may present as a different color from surrounding tissue; epidermis is intact
Stage 2	Partial-thickness; epidermis is missing; wound base is pink and moist
Stage 3	Full-thickness; epidermis and dermis is missing; wound base is generally yellow because hypodermis is exposed
Stage 4	Full-thickness; bone, muscle, and/or organs are identifiable in wound base
Unstageable	Eschar-covered area over a boney prominence that obscures identification of depth of tissue damage
Deep tissue injury	Presents as purple discolored area that may or may not evolve to full-thickness wound depth Epidermis is intact over this area
Medical device-related pressure ulcers	Partial- to full-thickness tissue damage related to a medical device (eg, wrongly positioned urinary catheter, endotracheal tube)

Data from WOCN Guideline for prevention and management of pressure ulcers (injuries). Philadelphia: WOCN; 2016; and Stechmiller JK, Cowan LJ, Oomens CWJ. Bottom-up (pressure shear) injuries. In Doughty DB, McNichol LL, editors. Wound, Ostomy, and Continence Nurses Society core curriculum: wound management. Philadelphia: Wolters Kluwer; 2016. p. 313–31.

Table 8
Impairment of lower extremity skin due to vascular-related issues

Disease Issue	Clinical Presentation	Treatment Focus
Arterial insufficiency ulcers or injuries	• Shallow wound • Minimal exudate • Lateral malleolus or foot area • May present as spontaneous blackened area • Increased pain with rest	• Nonconstrictive garments and dressings • Nonadherent dressings • Wound gel to add moisture • Prevention of additional trauma
Neuropathic ulcers or injuries	• Shallow or full-thickness wound • Minimal exudate • Plantar surface of foot • Callus may be present • Not associated with pain	• Wound gel to add moisture • Offloading foot orthotic or device • Nonadherent dressing • Regular follow-up with clinician to assure neuropathic issue is not worsening • Foot care education • Foot and nail care by experts only
Venous insufficiency ulcers or injuries	• Shallow wound • Moderate to large amounts of exudate • Medial malleolus or gaiter area • Periwound area and/or lower leg may have dermatitis with complaints of itching • Increased pain toward end of day • Edema from knee to foot area	• Compression therapy based on ankle-brachial index • Shallow wound • Minimal exudate • Lateral malleolus or foot area • May present as spontaneous blackened area • Increased pain with rest

Data from Refs.[1,17–20].

Recurrence of Venous Leg Ulcers, available online at http://vlu.wocn.org/#home.[17]
- WOCN *Guideline for Management of Wounds in Patients with Lower-Extremity Arterial Disease*[18]
- WOCN *Guideline for Management of Wounds in Patients with Lower-Extremity Neuropathic Disease*[19]
- WOCN *Guideline for Management of Wounds in Patients with Lower-Extremity Venous Disease*[20]
- WOCN *Core Curriculum: Wound Management.*[1]

Cancer

Cancer lesions, such as basal-cell carcinoma, can occur as a normal process within skin aging.[1,2] Larger cancer lesions and skin damage related to chemotherapeutic medications and/or radiation therapy also present challenges for treatment. Many larger lesions, also named fungating tumors, are highly vascular but also contain necrotic tissues. Copious amounts of drainage and foul odor are common issues with many of these wounds. Using charcoal-impregnated dressings or medication-impregnated dressings may help with the odor. Gentle wound care and absorptive dressing options are a must. As previously mentioned, an underlying fungal skin infection may also be present and require additional treatment using antifungal agents. Containment of odor and control of pain can improve the individual's quality of life. Given the location of many tumors, creative dressing application techniques may be required.

OTHER CAUSES OF IMPAIRMENT IN SKIN INTEGRITY

Feeding tubes and other percutaneous tubes, intravenous tubes, chest tubes, and other medical-related drain tubes cause impairment in skin integrity. Surgical incisions and fistula formation (enterocutaneous, esophagocutaneous, and others) are also categorized as impairments in skin integrity. All percutaneous tubes should be stabilized to reduce excessive manipulation and prevent erosion.[1] When erosion occurs, body fluids creep onto the skin and cause increased risk for impairment and infection. Containing the drainage (eg, mucus, gastric) and protecting the skin from excess moisture is critical to maintaining health skin tissue.[1]

SUMMARY

Management of skin tissue impairment is more than just managing a wound. A comprehensive assessment of the individual's health (particularly diabetes), nutrition (eg, protein, vitamins), comorbidities, and activity levels are key to formulating the best treatment plan for the individual.[1] Positive outcomes for the elderly involves a team approach: medical team, family team, and others. Involving experts and using evidence-based resources readily available online will also improve patient outcomes and assure quality of life for the elderly.

REFERENCES

1. Doughty D. Emory University Wound, Ostomy, and Continence Nursing Education Center's wound core curriculum. Atlanta (GA): Emory University WOCNEC; 2016. p. 1–312.
2. Mufti A, Ayello EA, Sibbald RG. Anatomy and physiology of the skin. In: Doughty DB, McNichol LL, editors. Wound, Ostomy, and Continence Nurses

Society core curriculum: wound management. Philadelphia: Wolters Kluwer; 2016. p. 3–23.

3. Weschler CJ. Squalene and cholesterol in dust from Danish homes and daycare centers. Environ Sci Technol 2011;45:3872–9.
4. Schleicher SM. Skin Sense!: a dermatologist's guide to skin and facial care. 3rd Edition. Bloomington (IN): iUniverse; 2015.
5. Westra BL, Bliss DZ, Savik K, et al. Effectiveness of wound, ostomy, and continence nurses on agency-level wound and incontinence outcomes in home care. J Wound Ostomy Continence Nurs 2013;40(16):25–53.
6. Strazzieri-Pulido KC, Peres GRP, Campanili TCGF, et al. Skin tear prevalence and associated factors: a systematic review. Rev Esc Enferm USP 2015;49(4):0674–80. Available at: http://www.scielo.br/scielo.php?script=sci_arttext&pid=S0080-62342015000400674&lng=en&nrm=iso. Accessed May 31, 2017.
7. International Skin Tear Advisory Panel. Available at: http://www.skintears.org. Accessed December 28, 2016.
8. LeBlanc K, Baranoski S, Christensen D, et al. International Skin Tear Advisory Panel: a tool kit to aid in the prevention, assessment, and treatment of skin tears using a simplified classification system. Adv Skin Wound Care 2013;26:459–76.
9. McNichol LL, Lund C, Rosen T, et al. Medical adhesives and patient safety: state of the science: consensus statements for the assessment, prevention, and treatment of adhesive-related skin injuries. Orthop Nurs 2013;32(5):267–81.
10. Kennedy-Evans K, Smith DR, Viggiano B, et al. Multisite feasibility study using a new textile with silver for management of skin conditions located in skin folds. J Wound Ostomy Continence Nurs 2007;34(3S):S68.
11. National Pressure Ulcer Advisory Panel. Available at: http://www.npuap.org. Accessed December 28, 2016.
12. WOCN® Guideline for prevention and management of pressure ulcers (injuries). Philadelphia: WOCN; 2016.
13. Braden scale for predicting pressure sore risk. Available at: http://www.bradenscale.com. Accessed December 28, 2016.
14. Stechmiller JK, Cowan LJ, Oomens CWJ. Bottom-up (pressure shear) injuries. In: Doughty DB, McNichol LL, editors. Wound, Ostomy, and Continence Nurses Society core curriculum: wound management. Philadelphia: Wolters Kluwer; 2016. p. 313–31.
15. Maklebust JA, Magnan MA. Pressure ulcer prevention: specific measures and agency-wide strategies. In: Doughty DB, McNichol LL, editors. Wound, Ostomy, and Continence Nurses Society core curriculum: wound management. Philadelphia: Wolters Kluwer; 2016. p. 333–61.
16. WOCN® support surface algorithm. Available at: http://algorithm.wocn.org/#home. Accessed December 28, 2016.
17. WOCN® compression for primary prevention, treatment and prevention of recurrence of venous leg ulcers algorithm. Available at: http://vlu.wocn.org/#home. Accessed December 28, 2016.
18. WOCN® Guideline for management of wounds in patients with lower-extremity arterial disease. Philadelphia: WOCN; 2014.
19. WOCN® guideline for management of wounds in patients with lower-extremity neuropathic disease. Philadelphia: WOCN; 2012.
20. WOCN® Guideline for management of wounds in patients with lower-extremity venous disease. Philadelphia: WOCN; 2015.

Gastrointestinal Disturbances in the Elderly

Natalie R. Baker, DNP, ANP-BC, GNP-BC[a],*, Kala K. Blakely, DNP, NP-C[b]

KEYWORDS

- Gastrointestinal • Older adults • Age-related changes • Dysphagia • GERD
- GI bleeding • Colorectal cancer screening

KEY POINTS

- The aging process impacts how the gastrointestinal (GI) system digests, absorbs and excretes nutrients and medications and disrupts GI immunity responses.
- All older adults will exhibit some degree of swallowing difficulty, also known as senescent swallowing.
- Older adults may have nonspecific abdominal complaints that may require a thorough history and comprehensive physical examination, as well as prescription and over-the-counter medications.
- Older adults are prone to GI bleeding, gastroesophageal reflux disease, chronic gastritis, constipation, and cholelithiasis.
- Colorectal cancer screening tests should be discussed with all older adults due to the high incidence of colorectal cancer in this patient population.

INTRODUCTION

The gastrointestinal (GI) system is composed of a muscular tube extending from the mouth to anus and accessory digestive organs, which include the liver, gallbladder, and pancreas.[1–3] This muscular tube, also known as the alimentary tube,[4] is approximately 23 feet in length[2] and consists of the esophagus, stomach, and small and large intestines[1–3]; also included are the liver, gallbladder, and pancreas.[5] Recognized as a complex system, the GI tract is dependent on a coordinated network of organs, sphincters, and hormones, as well as enteric nervous, lymphatic, and circulatory systems to achieve its primary responsibility: providing the body with nutrients.[1–4]

The 4 functions of the GI system are digestion, absorption, excretion, and immune defense.[1,3,4] Nutrients and medications are digested through a series of mechanical

The authors have nothing to disclose.
[a] School of Nursing, University of Alabama at Birmingham, NB 536, 1720 2nd Avenue South, Birmingham, AL 35294-1210, USA; [b] School of Nursing, University of Alabama at Birmingham, 528C, 1720 2nd Avenue South, Birmingham, AL 35294-1210, USA
* Corresponding author.
E-mail address: nrbaker@uab.edu

and chemical processes, ultimately reducing the particles to molecules that are absorbed into the circulatory and lymphatic systems and eliminating nonabsorbable particles through the large intestines.[1,3,4] Within the mucosa of the GI tract are lymph nodules containing lymphocytes for immunologic response to bacteria that cross epithelial tissue.[4] The largest accumulation of tissue macrophages in the body is located within liver sinusoids. These phagocytic cells, including Kupffer cells, are bactericidal and vital for our innate immunity responses.[3]

The GI tract is impacted by the aging process, with some organs and functions more adversely impacted than others (**Table 1**). Effects of chronic disease and sustained use of alcohol, tobacco, and medications often exacerbate GI dysfunction exhibited by older adults.[5]

AGING CHANGES IN THE GASTROINTESTINAL TRACT
Oropharyngeal

Beginning with common age-related dentition issues, many older adults are plagued with chewing and swallowing issues. Poor dentition, coupled with xerostomia,[3,5,6] often requires changing the consistency of the food before mastication and deglutition can occur.[7] Some degree of oral motor dysfunction can be expected as one ages, and may contribute to the reason that older adults tend to swallow larger-sized food bites.[6] Difficulty with the mechanics of swallowing begins to occur in adults age 45 and older.

Table 1
Age-related gastrointestinal changes

Gastrointestinal Tract	Age-Related Change
Oropharynx	Dental decay Decreased saliva production Reduced chewing effectiveness Presbyphagia
Esophagus	Decreased upper esophageal sphincter pressure Decreased contractile amplitude during peristalsis Incomplete relaxation of lower esophageal sphincter Esophageal dilation
Stomach	Decreased motility Delayed emptying of liquids Decreased acid and pepsin production Increased gastrin production Decreased gastric mucosal cytoprotective factors
Small intestines	Decreased absorption[a] Decreased motility Decreased blood flow
Colon	Decreased motility Ineffective muscular contractions Decreased tensile strength and increased collagen in colon wall
Gallbladder	Altered chemical composition of bile Decreased emptying
Liver	Decreased size Decreased blood flow and perfusion
Pancreas	Decreased size Increased fibrosis and fatty acid deposits

[a] Vitamins B_{12} and D, folic acid, calcium, copper, zinc, fatty acids, cholesterol.
Adapted from Refs.[3,5,6]

Known as senescent swallowing or presbyphagia, all older adults will exhibit some degree of impaired deglutition. The term, dysphagia, is used when an individual has significant impairment in moving the food or fluid from the oropharynx to the esophagus or from the esophagus to the stomach.[8,9] Decreased oropharyngeal motility is frequently the result of neurologic disorders, such as cerebrovascular accident or dementia.[8,9]

The combination of weakened mastication ability and large size of food particles being pushed through to the esophagus from the oropharynx creates an anatomic and physiologic environment allowing for gastroesophageal-related aspiration.[10] Common complaints from patients with chewing or swallowing difficulties may include feeling as though food gets stuck when swallowing or a globus sensation, the urge to cough or feelings of choking on swallowing, and/or difficulty swallowing hard food items.[11] Older adults might notice a change in the sound quality of his or her voice.[12]

Assessment

In assessing these patients, dentition, oral cavity, throat, and neck should all be examined.[13] The severity of the symptoms can be determined using the volume-viscosity swallow test (V-VST). The V-VST will confirm chewing and swallowing difficulties through observability of impaired labial seal, oral or pharyngeal residue, and even piecemeal deglutition. Another sign of impaired swallowing ability is a decrease in oxygen saturation by 3% or greater when performing the V-VST.[12] In addition to physical swallowing assessments, laboratory values also should be monitored. Patients with chewing difficulties frequently have low levels of vitamin A, and if chewing and swallowing problems are present, decreased levels of vitamin E and magnesium are frequently observed.[14]

Prevention

Age-related oropharyngeal changes lead to a risk of aspiration due to weak upper esophageal sphincter pressure.[10] The key to preventing aspiration and treating oropharyngeal concerns relies on the clinician assessing the patient for pathophysiological changes along with monitoring the patient's nutritional status. It is incumbent on the provider to monitor the elderly patient's nutritional well-being and implement dietary modifications that adjust for the level of chewing and swallowing difficulties. The clinician should keep in mind that dietary intake of calories, protein, and other essential nutrients should be frequently assessed and maintained to prevent malnutrition related to oropharyngeal changes.[14]

Esophageal

Esophageal structure is only minimally affected by aging; however, its ability to propel nutrients and fluid into the stomach is frequently altered by underlying disease.[3,5] In most older adults experiencing dysphagia, the dysfunction is occurring in the esophagus.[9,15] As the food bolus distends through the esophagus, the flow is interrupted by uncoordinated peristaltic waves and increased lower esophageal sphincter tone. Subsequently, there is delayed passage of food into the stomach.[5] Correlation of clinical symptoms with age-related changes is only 20% to 30%; therefore, underlying diabetes, neurologic disorders, or medication adverse effects appear to be the primary culprits of esophageal dysfunction.[5]

Gastroesophageal reflux disease (GERD) symptoms are triggered by the reflux of stomach contents back into the esophagus. This disease is found in approximately one-fifth of the US population and presents itself with specific and nonspecific signs.[10] Clinical presentation can be very specific, with complaints such as a stomachache or stomach pain, hunger pains in the belly, heartburn, acid reflux, nausea, bloated stomach, and burping.[16] Other symptoms can be more vague, such as anorexia, weight loss, vomiting, dysphagia, coughing, wheezing, chest pain, and even enamel erosion of the teeth.[16,17] A thorough abdominal examination should be performed to assess for any areas of tenderness, as it is common for epigastric tenderness to be present with GERD.[13] A physical examination of the cardiac and pulmonary systems and nose and throat can assist with identifying differential diagnoses that present with similar symptoms as GERD but elicit different examination findings (**Table 2**).[13] Diagnostic testing is not needed for mild symptoms, especially if the symptoms are relieved by treatment recommendations. Upper endoscopy is recommended for patients with persistent symptoms after following GERD management protocols.[18] Most patients diagnosed with GERD can be managed with lifestyle changes and medication (**Table 3**).[10,18,19] Laparoscopic antireflux surgery is an option for patients with severe GERD that do not have relief of symptoms with lifestyle modifications and pharmacologic treatment.[19]

Gastric Function

Although considered part of the GI tube,[1–3] the stomach is a small hollow organ that serves as a food reservoir.[3] Gastric enzymes and peristaltic contractions partially digest food particles as they progress through the 3 sections of the stomach; a process that can last up to 6 hours.[3] Delayed gastric emptying allows caustic agents,

Table 2
Nonspecific symptoms with differential diagnoses

Symptoms	Differential Diagnosis or Common Causes
Anorexia, unintended weight loss	GERD Nutrient malabsorption
Vomiting	GERD Gastroenteritis Small bowel obstruction
Dysphagia	GERD Hiatal hernia Barrett esophagus
Coughing	GERD Allergic rhinitis Medication side effect (such as ACE inhibitors) Pulmonary: asthma, COPD, bronchitis
Wheezing	GERD Pulmonary: asthma, COPD, bronchitis
Chest pain	GERD Myocardial infarction Angina
Dentition changes	GERD Poor dental hygiene Tobacco use

Abbreviations: ACE, angiotensin-converting enzyme; COPD, chronic obstructive pulmonary disease; GERD, gastroesophageal reflux disease.

Adapted from Pilotto A, Maggi S, Noale M, Franceschi M, Parisi G, Crepaldi G. Association of upper gastrointestinal symptoms with functional and clinical characteristics in the elderly. World J Gastroenterol 2011;17(25):3020–6; and Patti MG. Gastroesophageal reflux disease. Medscape. http://www.emedicine.medscape.com/article/176595. Accessed November 10, 2016.

Table 3	
Gastroesophageal reflux disease treatment options	
Management Method	**Options**
Nonpharmacologic (lifestyle changes)	Decrease acidic food intake Minimal caffeine consumption Weight reduction for overweight patients Elevate head of bed Refrain from eating 2–3 h before sleep
Pharmacologic	Proton pump inhibitors (first-line therapy) Histamine-2 antagonists Over-the-counter antacids
Surgical	Laparoscopic antireflux surgery

Adapted from Refs.[10,18,19]

such as nonsteroidal anti-inflammatory drugs (NSAIDs), prolonged contact with the mucosal lining, thereby increasing the risk of mucosal injury. Additionally, increased exposure to NSAIDs while in the stomach further reduces cytoprotective factors, such as mucosal prostaglandins.[5]

Atrophic gastritis

Older adults are prone to chronic gastritis, also referred to as atrophic gastritis, resulting in chronic inflammation, mucosal atrophy and epithelial metaplasia.[3] Atrophic gastritis is associated with *Helicobacter pylori*[20] and decreased secretion of intrinsic factor that is vital for vitamin B12 absorption in the small intestines.[3]

Atrophic gastritis and autoimmune gastritis are both sequelae of *H pylori* and/or malabsorption of vitamin B12 and iron.[21,22] Clinical presentation of gastritis often begins with dyspeptic symptoms; however, this is not age specific.[22] Patients may complain of nausea that is not attributed to diet, change in medications, or any known structural changes. These symptoms are often persistent for more than 6 months.[13] Laboratory work for geriatric patients frequently show vitamin B12 and iron deficiency. Similar to patients with GERD, it is imperative that the clinician perform a thorough abdominal examination to assess for epigastric pain. Gastritis is confirmed with an endoscopy (**Box 1** for endoscopy indications).[23] Endoscopy allows for further

Box 1
Clinical recommendations for endoscopy

- 50 years of age

- Gastrointestinal (GI) bleeding

- Iron deficiency

- Dysphagia

- Persistent vomiting

- Unintentional weight loss

- Pain in mouth or esophagus with swallowing

- Family history of upper GI malignancy

Adapted from Shaukat A, Wang A, Acosta RD, et al. The role of endoscopy in dyspepsia. Gastrointest Endosc 2015; 82(2):227–32.

investigation of patient symptoms and provides an internal view of the severity of gastric inflammation. Patients with persistent symptoms of dyspepsia also should be assessed for delayed gastric emptying.[22]

Treatment for gastritis should include treating the underlying cause of gastritis, such as H pylori and B12 replacement. It is crucial to educate patients on decreasing the use or avoidance of NSAIDs to prevent recurrence of gastritis in the future. Early diagnosis and treatment of H pylori and B12 deficiency also can serve as prevention of gastritis.[22]

Upper gastrointestinal bleeding

Following mucosal changes from gastritis and peptic ulcers, upper gastrointestinal bleeding (UGIB) has unfortunately been a common occurrence among the elderly (**Table 4** for common causes of GI bleeding). The cardinal sign of UGIB is the clinical presentation of hematemesis. Patients may report vomiting that is the consistency and color of coffee grounds and/or melena.[24] It is time sensitive for the clinician to assess the hemodynamic stability of patients. Signs of hypovolemia, such as hypotension, tachycardia, and hemoglobin less than 8 g/dL at initial presentation are significant signs that a patient should have fluid losses corrected immediately.[24] Crystalloid intravenous fluids, like lactate ringer, supplemental oxygen, and transfusion of packed red blood cells, are all used to resuscitate the patient's fluid volume.[24] Once the patient is hemodynamically stable, endoscopy can be performed immediately to determine the cause of bleeding, potentially stop the bleeding, and offer prognostic details.[25] Future prevention of UGIB includes use of a proton pump inhibitor to reduce risk of rebleeding.[26]

Small Intestines

Measuring an estimated 1 inch (2.5 cm) in diameter and 20 feet (6 m) in length, the functions of absorption and GI immunity primarily occur in the small intestines.[4] Despite some age-related changes in the small intestines, significant effects are not observed without the presence of additional nonaging pathology.[5] However, older adults do tend to exhibit decreased levels of some vitamins and nutrients due to decreased small intestine absorption.[5] There have been some studies that suggest aging effects on the small intestines also results in decreased absorption of protein and carbohydrates.[3,5]

Small bowel obstruction (SBO) often presents as acute, diffuse abdominal pain and vomiting unrelated to a change in diet. It is most commonly associated with adhesions from recent surgery, Crohn disease, abdominal neoplasms, and hernias.[27] A detailed

Table 4 Common causes for GI bleeding	
Upper GI Bleeding	**Lower GI Bleeding**
NSAIDs	NSAIDs
Aspirin	Aspirin
Anticoagulants	Diverticular disease
Gastritis	Ischemic colitis
Peptic Ulcers	Angiodysplasia
Esophagitis	Colonic neoplasms
	Hemorrhoids

Abbreviations: GI, gastrointestinal; NSAID, nonsteroidal anti-inflammatory drug.
Adapted from Refs.[25,34,46]

medical history sets the foreground of what the contributing factor is for the patient's presentation. On physical examination, the clinician likely will find diffuse abdominal tenderness to palpation and possibly generalized peritonitis.[28] These patients should be evaluated for signs of systemic toxicity, such as fever, continuous pain, leukocytosis, tachycardia, and metabolic acidosis.[28] Radiography is most often used to determine if an obstruction is present. If SBO is suspected, use of computed tomography is preferred for confirmation, along with determining the degree of the dilatation.[27] Patients with signs of systemic toxicity, complete obstruction, strangulation, or bowel perforation are candidates for immediate surgical repair. For those with less severe symptoms, nonsurgical evaluation, such as inpatient monitoring, should take place to ensure resolution. Contrast studies should be performed if the SBO has not resolved within 48 hours.[28]

Colon

Unlike inconsequential aging effects in the small intestines, the colon (large intestines) exhibits significant age-related alterations.[5] The colon, measuring an estimated 2.5 inches (6.3 cm) in diameter and 5 feet (1.5 m) in length is the last opportunity for the GI system to absorb nutrients and fluids before indigestible residue is excreted.[3,4] Once the nutrients and fluids enter the cecum (beginning section of colon), the average length of time it will take these substances to travel to the rectum is 1 to 2 days in healthy adults.[1] Age-induced decreased colonic motility extends the time that the substances are traveling through the colon, although constipation has not definitely been linked to this phenomenon.[5] However, ineffective age-related muscular contractions appear to increase the colon's resorption of water, thus producing hard feces.[5] Although fecal incontinence is more prevalent in older adults compared with the general population, it is not the result of the normal aging process.[5]

Diverticulosis
It is postulated that diverticulosis is the result of age-related changes within the colon wall.[5] Given the increased prevalence of colon cancer in older adults, it is possible that the normal aging colon may be susceptible to the oncogenic effects of growth factors and carcinogens.[5] Due to the sharp curvature of the colon, it is not uncommon for digestive products to build up in the pockets of the colon. Diverticulosis clinical presentation varies between patients and is often diagnosed by ruling out other conditions.[29] The symptoms might include abdominal pain and changes in bowel habits, such as constipation. A physical examination may or may not reveal abdominal tenderness in the left lower quadrant. Due to the varying nature of presentation, abdominal examination alone does not serve as a diagnosis confirmation for diverticulosis.[29] Colonoscopy is the diagnostic tool of choice in verifying the cause of the abdominal pain. Along with educating patients on foods to avoid that cause a buildup within the diverticulum, in the past, probiotics have been the medication most frequently prescribed for treatment of diverticulosis.[29]

Constipation
Elderly patients commonly present with complaints of constipation as a result of the colon's resorption of water.[5,30] Occasional constipation has been reported by one-third of adults age 60 or older.[31] The symptoms include incomplete elimination of stool and/or difficulty passing stool. Constipation can be the result of a primary cause related to physiologic changes or a secondary factor, such as medication use.[30] Diagnosis of constipation can be confirmed based on symptomatic presentation. It is important to assess the patient for any underlying causes, such as chronic diseases,

neoplasms, or impaction. Fecal impaction can be determined by performing a rectal examination.[30] The treatment goal for these patients is to reduce stool hardness and increase stool frequency without causing diarrhea. Nonpharmacological management of constipation includes encouraging adequate water intake, consumption of 20 to 35 g of fiber per day, and consistent toileting times. Those requiring further management may benefit from use of a laxative, such as polyethylene glycol, to increase bowel movement frequency. Psyllium also can be used to assist with softening the stool for those with more difficulty passing stool.[30]

Hemorrhoids

Hemorrhoids often present symptoms of bright red blood covering stool, on tissue after wiping or small drips of blood in the toilet after defecation. Hemorrhoids can be internal, in which the thrombosis remains within the anal canal, or external, in which the thrombosis protrudes from the anus.[32] A digital rectal examination and anoscopy can assist with ruling out differential diagnoses, such as skin tags, anal fissure, perianal dermatitis, and rectal mass.[33] Sitz baths, regular exercise, low-fat diet, proper hydration, and adequate fiber intake are all modalities of preventing hemorrhoids.[32] Patients are encouraged to decrease or eliminate activities that require straining, like heavy lifting or straining to defecate. To prevent straining when having difficulty passing stool, it is also important to review with patients medications that increase the risk of constipation.[32] Hemorrhoids that persistently cause unrelenting pain and continue to protrude often require surgical excision.[32]

Lower gastrointestinal bleeding

Lower gastrointestinal bleeding (LGIB) is defined as any blood loss that occurs distal to the ligament of Treitz (see **Table 4** for common causes of GI bleeding).[34] Clinical presentation can include complaints of change in bowel habits, hematochezia, and rectal or anal bleeding. A complete blood count may reveal anemia.[34] Along with an abdominal physical examination, a thorough history should be collected for concerns of underlying causes of the LGIB. In discussing aging effects of the large intestines, numerous diagnoses can lead to LGIB. Management of LGIB includes maintaining hemodynamic stability for those anemic or hypovolemic patients through transfusions. LGIB often spontaneously resolves; however, those that persist should undergo further diagnostic testing to determine the underlying cause.[34]

Colorectal cancer

Almost 60% of patients with colorectal cancer (CRC) are age 65 or older.[35] Clinical presentation of CRC is often asymptomatic; therefore, preventive screening is the key to early diagnosis and treatment. National CRC screening guidelines differ slightly (**Table 5**). The US Preventive Services Task Force (USPSTF) recommends CRC screening for all individuals age 50 to 75 and that for individuals age 76 to 85, decisions for screening be based on the individual's health and prior screening history. USPSTF guidelines recommend against screening for all individuals age 86 or older.[36] The American Cancer Society (ACS) and American College of Gastroenterology (ACG) do not recommend that CRC screening be discontinued based solely on an individual's age.[37,38] The ACS outlines acceptable screening modalities based on 2 categories: testing for polyps and cancer, and testing for cancer.[37] Guidelines established by the ACG have similar classifications as ACS but use different terminology: cancer prevention (potential to detect cancer and polyps) and cancer detection (tests that have low probability for detecting polyps and somewhat lower ability to detect cancer).[38] The clinician and patient should discuss which method of screening

Table 5
Colorectal cancer screening for average-risk individuals

USPSTF	American Cancer Society	American College of Gastroenterology
Age 50–75	*Age 50+*	*Age 50+ (Age 45+ African Americans)*
Stool Based	**Detection of Polyps and Cancer**	**Preferred Screening Tests**
gFOBT: q1 y	Flexible sigmoidoscopy:	**Cancer prevention**
FIT: q1 y	q5 y[a]	Colonoscopy: q10 y
Stool DNA test: q1–3 y	Double-contrast barium	Cancer detection: FIT:
Direct Visualization	enema: q5 y[a]	q1 y if
Colonoscopy: q10 y	CT Colonography: q5 y[a]	Colonoscopy or other
CT colonography: q5 y	Colonoscopy: q10 y	cancer prevention
Flexible sigmoidoscopy:	**Detection of Cancer**	test declined
q5 y	Stool DNA test: q3 y[a]	Alternative Prevention
Flexible sigmoidoscopy	gFOBT: q1 y[b]	Tests
with FIT: q5 y plus FIT	FIT: q1 y[b]	Flexible sigmoidoscopy:
q1 y		q5–10 y
Age 76–85		CT colonography: q5 y
Screening is individual		**Alternative Detection Tests**
decision based on health		Hemoccult sensa: q1 y
and prior screening		Stool DNA test: q3 y
history		
Age 86+		
Recommends against		
screening		

Abbreviations: FIT, fecal immunochemical test; gFOBT, guaiac-based fecal occult blood test; q, every; USPSTF, US Preventive Services Task Force.
[a] If results positive, patient should have colonoscopy.
[b] Highly sensitive versions of take-home multiple-sample method should be done. FIT or gFOBT done in clinic after digital rectal examination is not sufficient for cancer screening.
Adapted from Refs.[36–38]

is the best option for individualized patients. Treatment for CRC can include a single or combination of surgery, chemotherapy, or radiation.[39]

Hepatobiliary and Pancreas

An observed 30% to 40% decline in liver size, blood flow, and perfusion is noted between the third and tenth decades of life.[5] However, abnormal liver function tests, such as alkaline phosphatase and aminotransferases, are not related to these aging process,[3,5,40] and most hepatic abnormalities present in older adults are the result of comorbidities, genetics, or lifestyle choices (diet, alcohol, tobacco).[5] Age-induced decline in hepatic enzymes and blood flow does decrease metabolism of alcohol[3] and drugs that are dependent on the P450 system.[3,5,40–42] Once injured, the aging liver has a diminished capacity to regenerate.[42]

It is unclear if gallbladder function is altered as a result of aging, but the prevalence of cholelithiasis does increase with age and it appears the common bile duct may dilate with advanced age, although this has not been proven.[42] Although the pancreas does undergo some age-related structural changes, its digestive function is relatively unaltered.[3,5]

Cholelithiasis

Patients with cholelithiasis are frequently asymptomatic. For those with symptoms, clinical presentation may include severe upper abdominal pain that ranges from episodic to steady and lasts longer than 30 minutes. Associated symptoms include nausea with vomiting and possibly pain that radiates from the abdomen into the upper back.[43] In reviewing history with patients; ethnicity plays an important role in determining the type of gallstone that is more prevalent for a patient. Other nonmodifiable risks are being female, aging, and genetics. Those at high risk for cholelithiasis due to nonmodifiable risk factors can make changes in their diet and physical activity to prevent further risks such as obesity, diabetes, dyslipidemia, minimal physical activity, rapid weight loss, or unhealthy diet.[43] Ultrasound can be used to determine presence of gallstones. Patients with gallstones that are nonobstructing are monitored to determine whether the symptoms outweigh the risks and need for cholecystectomy. It is preferred to not seek surgical intervention unless obstruction or biliary pain is severe enough to require removal of the gallbladder in an effort to relieve the biliary symptoms.[43]

Pancreatitis

Pancreatitis most often presents as severe left upper quadrant or epigastric pain that may radiate to the back, chest, or flanks.[44] Amylase and lipase should be monitored; these levels are generally 3 times the normal upper limit within a few hours of symptom onset.[44] A transabdominal ultrasound is also recommended for patients with suspected acute pancreatitis. A computed tomographic scan with contrast or MRI can be used for patients with unclear diagnosis or failure to improve within 72 hours of onset.[44] These patients should be monitored for hemodynamic stability and resuscitated with fluids if needed. Close monitoring for acute organ failure is of the essence and endoscopic retrograde cholangiopancreatography within 24 hours of hospital admission for patients with concurrent acute cholangitis allows the clinician to more closely examine the pancreatic and bile ducts for abnormalities.[44]

Gastrointestinal Immunity Response

Immunity response by the GI system is vital to protect the body against oral or fecal transmission of pathogens. Recognized as the largest immunologic organ,[5] the mucosal walls of the GI tract are filled with lymphocytes and other antigen receptor cells that are triggered on pathogen entry.[45] This mucosal immune response within the small intestines[5] develops a tolerance to the colonized microflora, placing older adults at increased risk for infection.[45] It is unclear what age-related processes trigger this immune tolerance.[45]

SUMMARY

Age-related changes to the GI system create alterations in the body's ability to digest, absorb, and excrete nutrients. Age-related decrease in hepatic enzymes and blood flow decreases one's metabolism of alcohol and medications dependent on the P450 system. Changes within the mucosal lining of the small intestines create an environment of colonization to microflora, hence the GI immunity response becomes blunted as a result of changes associated with the aging process. Effects of chronic disease and sustained use of alcohol, tobacco, and medications often exacerbates age-related GI dysfunction exhibited by older adults.

All older adults will exhibit some degree of swallowing difficulty, also known as senescent swallowing. Prone to common GI disorders, such as GI bleeding, GERD, atrophic gastritis, constipation, and cholelithiasis, older adults often have nonspecific complaints, warranting a thorough heath history, including prescription and over-the-counter medications, and comprehensive physical examination. Atrophic gastritis is associated with *H pylori* and decreased absorption of vitamin B12 and iron. Colorectal cancer screening tests should be discussed with all older adults due to the high incidence of colorectal cancer in this patient population.

REFERENCES

1. Barrett KE. Gastrointestinal physiology. 2nd edition. New York: McGraw-Hill Education; 2014.
2. Sartin JS. Gastrointestinal function. In: Copstead LC, Banasik JL, editors. Pathophysiology. 3rd edition. St Louis (MO): Elsevier Saunders; 2005. p. 860–86.
3. Doig AK, Huether SE. Structure and function of the digestive system. In: McCance KL, Huether SE, editors. Pathophysiology. 7th edition. St Louis (MO): Elsevier Mosby; 2014. p. 1393–422.
4. Scanlon VC, Sanders T. The digestive system. In: Scanlon VC, Sanders T, editors. Essentials of anatomy and physiology. 7th edition. Philadelphia: F.A. Davis Co; 2015. p. 408–35.
5. Hall KE. Effect of aging on gastrointestinal function. In: Halter JB, Ouslander JG, Tinetti ME, et al, editors. Hazzard's geriatric medicine and gerontology. 6th edition. New York: McGraw-Hill Companies, Inc.; 2009. p. 1059–64.
6. Ship JA. Oral cavity. In: Halter JB, Ouslander JG, Tinetti ME, et al, editors. Hazzard's geriatric medicine and gerontology. 6th edition. New York: McGraw-Hill Companies, Inc.; 2009. p. 501–10.
7. Shay K. Dental and oral disorders. In: Duthie EH, Katz PR, Malone ML, editors. Practice of geriatrics. 4th edition. Philadelphia: Saunders Elsevier; 2007. p. 547–61.
8. Robbins J, Hind J, Barczi S. Disorders of swallowing. In: Halter JB, Ouslander JG, Tinetti ME, et al, editors. Hazzard's geriatric medicine and gerontology. 6th edition. New York: McGraw-Hill Companies, Inc.; 2009. p. 483–99.
9. Hall KE. Gastrointestinal and abdominal complaints. In: Williams BA, Chang A, Ahalt C, et al, editors. Current diagnosis and treatment geriatrics. 2nd edition. New York: McGraw-Hill Education; 2014. p. 244–55.
10. Achem SR, DeVault KR. Gastroesophageal reflux disease and the elderly. Gastroenterol Clin North Am 2014;43:147–60.
11. Holland G, Jayasekeran V, Pendleton N, et al. Prevalence and symptom profiling of oropharyngeal dysphagia in a community dwelling of an elderly population: a self-reporting questionnaire survey. Dis Esophagus 2011;24:476–80.
12. Serra-Prat M, Palomera M, Gomez C, et al. Oropharyngeal dysphagia as a risk factor for malnutrition and lower respiratory tract infection in independently living older persons: a population-based prospective study. Age Ageing 2012;41(3): 376–81.
13. Bickley L. Bates' guide to physical examination and history-taking. 11th edition. Philadelphia: Lipincott Williams Wilkins; 2013.
14. Mann T, Heuberger R, Wong H. The association between chewing and swallowing difficulties and nutritional status in older adults. Aust Dent J 2013;58:200–6.
15. Pilotto A, Francheschi M. Upper gastrointestinal disorders. In: Halter JB, Ouslander JG, Tinetti ME, et al, editors. Hazzard's geriatric medicine and gerontology. 6th edition. New York: McGraw-Hill Companies, Inc.; 2009. p. 1075–90.
16. Pilotto A, Maggi S, Noale M, et al. Association of upper gastrointestinal symptoms with functional and clinical characteristics in the elderly. World J Gastroenterol 2011;17(25):3020–6.

17. Patti MG. Gastroesophageal reflux disease. Medscape. Available at: http://www.emedicine.medscape.com/article/176595. Accessed November 10, 2016.
18. Katz PO, Gerson LB, Vela MF. Guidelines for the diagnosis and management of gastroesophageal reflux disease. Am J Gastroenterol 2013;108:308–28.
19. Vela MF. Medical treatments of GERD. Gastroenterol Clin North Am 2014;43(1):121–33.
20. Fromm AL. Care of older adult populations diagnosed with *Helicobacter pylori*. Gastroenterol Nurs 2009;32(6):393–8.
21. Aine R, Kahar E, Aitokari K, et al. Atrophic gastritis (AG) and its clinical sequels among elderly people in Finland and Estonia. A comparative study using gastropanel and B12-vitamin testing of the residents in assisted-housing facilities. J Aging Res Clin Pract, in press.
22. Kalkan C, Soykan I. Differences between older and young patients with autoimmune gastritis. Geriatr Gerontol Int 2016;1–6.
23. Shaukat A, Wang A, Acosta RD, et al. The role of endoscopy in dyspepsia. Gastrointest Endosc 2015;82(2):227–32.
24. Khamaysi I, Gralnek IM. Acute upper gastrointestinal bleeding (UGIB)–initial evaluation and management. Best Pract Res Clin Gastroenterol 2013;27:633–8.
25. Lau JL, Barkun A, Fan D, et al. Challenges in the management of acute peptic ulcer bleeding. Lancet 2013;381:2033–43.
26. Leontiadis GI, Sreedharan A, Dorward S, et al. Systematic reviews of the clinical effectiveness and cost-effectiveness of proton pump inhibitors in acute upper gastrointestinal bleeding. Health Technol Assess 2007;11(51):1–164. Available at: https://www.ncbi.nlm.nih.gov/books/NBK56852/.
27. Mullan CP, Siewert B, Eisenberg RL. Small bowel obstruction. AJR Am J Roentgenol 2012;198:W105–17.
28. Maung AA, Johnson DC, Piper GL, et al. Evaluation and management of small-bowel obstruction: an Eastern Association for the Surgery of Trauma practice management guideline. J Trauma Acute Care Surg 2012;73(5):S362–9.
29. Tursi A, Picchio M, Elisei W, et al. Current management of patients with diverticulosis and diverticular disease. J Clin Gastroenterol 2016;50(1):S97–100.
30. Mounsey A, Raleigh M, Wilson A. Management of constipation in older adults. Am Fam Physician 2015;92(6):500–4. Available at: http://www.aafp.org/afp/2015/0915/p500.html.
31. Bharucha AE, Pemberton JH, Locke GR III. American Gastroenterological Association technical review on constipation. Gastroenterology 2013;144(1):218–38.
32. Moss AK, Bordeianou L. Outpatient management of hemorrhoids. Semin Colon Rectal Surg 2013;24:76–80.
33. Lohsiriwat V. Hemorrhoids: from basic pathophysiology to clinical management. World J Gastroenterol 2012;18(17):2009–17.
34. Zuccaro G. Epidemiology of lower gastrointestinal bleeding. Best Pract Res Clin Gastroenterol 2008;22(2):225–32.
35. McCleary NJ, Dotan E, Browner I. Refining the chemotherapy approach for older patients with colon cancer. J Clin Oncol 2014;32:2570–80.
36. US Preventive Services Task Force. Screening for colorectal cancer: US Preventive Services Task Force recommendation statement. JAMA 2016;315(23):2564–75.
37. American Cancer Society. Colorectal cancer prevention and early detection. Atlanta (GA): American Cancer Society; 2016. Available at: http://www.cancer.org/acs/groups/cid/documents/webcontent/003170-pdf.pdf. Accessed December 20, 2016.

38. Rex DK, Johnson DA, Anderson JC, et al. American College of Gastroenterology guidelines for colorectal cancer screening 2008. Am J Gastroenterol 2009;104: 739–50.
39. Hubbard JM. Management of colorectal cancer in older adults. Clin Geriatr Med 2016;32(1):97–111.
40. Dua KS, Shaker R, Koch TR, et al. Gastroenterologic disorders. In: Duthie EH, Katz PR, Malone ML, editors. Practice of geriatrics. 4th edition. Philadelphia: Saunders Elsevier; 2007. p. 577–605.
41. Hilmer SN, Ford GA. General principles of pharmacology. In: Halter JB, Ouslander JG, Tinetti ME, et al, editors. Hazzard's geriatric medicine and gerontology. 6th edition. New York: McGraw-Hill Companies, Inc.; 2009. p. 103–21.
42. Rice JC, Barancin C, Benson M, et al. Hepatic, biliary, and pancreatic disease. In: Halter JB, Ouslander JG, Tinetti ME, et al, editors. Hazzard's geriatric medicine and gerontology. 6th edition. New York: McGraw-Hill Companies, Inc.; 2009. p. 1065–73.
43. Stinton LM, Shaffer EA. Epidemiology of gallbladder disease: cholelithiasis and cancer. Gut Liver 2012;6(2):172–87.
44. Tenner S, Baillie J, DeWitt J, et al. American College of Gastroenterology guideline: management of acute pancreatitis. Am J Gastroenterol 2013;108:1400–15.
45. Weinberger B, Weiskopf D, Grubeck-Loebenstein B. Immunology and aging. In: Halter JB, Ouslander JG, Tinetti ME, et al, editors. Hazzard's geriatric medicine and gerontology. 6th edition. New York: McGraw-Hill Companies, Inc; 2009. p. 23–36.
46. Bounds BC, Kelsey PB. Lower GI bleeding. Gastrointest Endosc Clin N Am 2007; 17(2):273–88. Available at: https://www.clinicalkey.com/#!/content/playContent/1-s2.0-S1052515707000281?returnurl=null&referrer=null.

Nutritional Problems Affecting Older Adults

Neva L. Crogan, PhD, ARNP, GNP-BC, ACHPN, FNGNA

KEYWORDS

- Malnutrition • Anorexia of aging • Sarcopenia • Cachexia • Dehydration
- Oral health

KEY POINTS

- Only those older adults with an actual deficiency determined by a laboratory blood test should be treated with an oral supplement.
- Successful treatment of depression can reverse weight loss in older adults.
- Hypernatremia and hyponatremia are the most common electrolyte abnormalities found in older adults and both are associated with a high mortality.

INTRODUCTION

Food and water are basic to life. For the older adult, food means family, togetherness, and quality of life. In older age there are physiologic changes resulting from a decrease in energy needs and expenditures referred to as anorexia of aging.[1] This physiologic anorexia results from changes related to normal aging, such as alterations in taste and smell and earlier satiation.[2] Nurses need to be able to successfully identify, evaluate, and treat problems affecting food and fluid intake and nutritional status. This article describes potential nutritional problems affecting older adults and then discusses evidence-based assessment strategies and treatment modalities that target these problems.

MALNUTRITION

Anorexia of aging is a physiologic process that occurs with older age. This physiologic anorexia increases the risk of developing weight loss and malnutrition when an older adult develops a physical or psychological illness.[1] Malnutrition is defined as "the state of being poorly nourished"[3(p4)] and can be caused by a lack of nutrients (undernutrition) or an excess of nutrients (overnutrition). For the older adult, the cause is usually a lack of nutrients, or undernutrition. The prevalence of malnutrition in community

Disclosure Statement: The author has nothing to disclose.
Department of Nursing, Gonzaga University, 502 East Boone Avenue, Spokane, WA 99258, USA
E-mail address: crogan@gonzaga.edu

Nurs Clin N Am 52 (2017) 433–445
http://dx.doi.org/10.1016/j.cnur.2017.04.005

nursing.theclinics.com

dwelling older adults is 15%; if homebound, the prevalence is variable at 5% to 44%.[4] The prevalence among those living in nursing homes is 30% to 85%,[4,5] and 20% to 60% if hospitalized.[4]

Sarcopenia and cachexia are two major markers of malnutrition in older adults.[6] Sarcopenia is defined as "a syndrome of progressive and generalized loss of skeletal muscle mass and strength, which increases the risk of adverse outcomes, such as physical disability, poor quality of life, and even death."[7(p20)] A clinical presentation of decreased muscle mass and either decreased physical performance or decreased muscle strength confirms a diagnosis of sarcopenia. Cachexia is a complex metabolic process associated with an underlying terminal illness (eg, end-stage renal disease, cancer) and is characterized by loss of fat and muscle mass, and anorexia.[2] Cachexia usually presents with severe wasting and is frequently associated with insulin resistance, breakdown of muscle protein, and inflammation. Of interest, older adults who present with cachexia also have sarcopenia, but those with sarcopenia frequently do not have cachexia.[7]

MICRONUTRIENT DEFICIENCY

Vitamin and mineral supplements are commonly recommended for older adults. However, supplementation may not be the best approach. The best way to ingest micronutrients is to eat a well-balanced diet. If this is not possible, supplementation may be needed. However, only those older adults with an actual deficiency determined by a laboratory blood test should be treated with an oral supplement.

For older adults living in the community (nursing homes, assisted living facilities, or group homes), oral nutritional supplements may not be the best first approach. Fortified foods, or those foods chosen based on their enhancement during processing (with vitamins and minerals) or enhanced with butter or cream during preparation, were found to be the best first approach to improving food intake and health in this population.[8]

IMPLICATIONS

A lack of food or nutrients affects most organ systems.[4] Malnutrition can lead to delayed wound healing, the development of pressure ulcers, increased susceptibility to infections, delayed recovery from acute illness, functional decline, cognitive decline and depression,[4] difficulty in swallowing, and dehydration.[2]

Malnutrition also can result in decreased lean body mass, lessened muscular strength and aerobic capacity, and alterations in gait and balance, increasing the risk for falls and fractures. For many older adults, this progression of events leads to frailty, dependence, and decreased quality of life.[2] Often used as a measure of malnutrition, body mass index is an easy-to-use measure of body fat levels and is determined using the calculation in **Box 1**.[4]

FACTORS INFLUENCING NUTRITIONAL RISK

Many factors contribute to weight loss and malnutrition in older adults. These factors are classified into three major groups: (1) social, (2) psychological, and (3) biologic

---

Box 1
Body mass index

Body mass index (BMI) is a useful measurement for malnutrition and is calculated using the following formula: BMI = weight (kg)/height (m^2)

(**Table 1**).[7] Furthermore, there are several medications associated with poor appetite and weight loss (**Box 2**).[3]

NUTRITIONAL ASSESSMENT

Nutritional risk screening is an integral part of the comprehensive assessment.[9] Many screening methods are available, including specific clinical screening tools (**Box 3**), anthropometric and body composition measurements (**Box 4**), laboratory tests (**Box 5**), a review of clinical data, and examination of an individual's diet history. Each method has strengths and weaknesses, thus a combination of approaches is best.[7]

Clinical Data Review

Clinical data specific to nutritional assessment in older adults includes a review of current medications, evaluation of oral and swallowing problems, review of gastrointestinal problems, and a review of psychiatric and neurologic disorders.[9]

Diet History Review

The final component of the nutritional assessment is an evaluation of the older adult's diet history. There are numerous strategies that could be used to complete a diet history review. For example, the health care provider could conduct a 24-hour recall or the older adult could be asked to keep a food diary.[17] Either of these strategies is effective in completing a diet history review.

Table 1 Factors influencing nutritional risk	
Social • Isolation • Loneliness • Poverty • Dependency	Examples • Social isolation, loneliness, and grieving because of death of spouse. • Affording expensive medication on a limited income. • Inability to cook or shop for themselves. • Inability to feed self.
Psychological • Depression • Anxiety • Dementia • Bereavement	Examples • Depressed older adults may suffer from weakness (61%), stomach pains (37%), nausea (27%), anorexia (22%), and diarrhea (20%)[2] • Older adults with dementia can forget or refuse to eat. • Older adults with dementia may develop apraxia of swallowing and must be reminded to swallow. • Profound loss, leading to grief and prolonged bereavement, can lead to weight loss.
Biologic • Dentition • Loss of taste or smell • Gastrointestinal disorders • Muscle weakness • Dry mouth • Olfaction • Renal disease • Physical disability • Chronic obstructive pulmonary disease • Drug interactions	Examples • Diseases, such as stroke, tremors, or arthritis, may affect an older adult's ability to prepare or eat food. • Infections may result in confusion, anorexia, and negative nitrogen balance.[4] • Older adults with chronic obstructive pulmonary disease may have difficulty eating because of dyspnea. • Hyperthyroidism and Parkinson disease cause hypermetabolism, which can lead to weight loss. • Many medications cause anorexia leading to weight loss.

Box 2
Medications associated with weight loss

- Digoxin
- Theophylline
- Metformin
- Antibiotics
- Nonsteroidal anti-inflammatory drugs
- Psychotropic drugs: Prozac (fluoxetine), Lithium, phenothiazines

---

EVIDENCE-BASED STRATEGIES TO IMPROVE NUTRITION

- Dietary supplementation should not be routinely recommended, but rather used only to treat symptomatic nutrient deficiency disease.
- The consumption of food is always preferable to meal replacements or supplementation. If this is not possible or realistic, between-meal snacks or liquid caloric supplements can increase energy intake.[2]

Box 3
Nutritional assessment methods

Clinical Screening Tools
  Mini Nutritional Assessment
- A simple and reliable tool for assessing nutrition status in older adults.
- An 18-item questionnaire that takes 10 to 15 minutes to administer.
- A score between 8 and 11 indicates an increased risk for malnutrition, and a score <7 reflects malnutrition.[7]
- A shortened version includes six items and takes <5 minutes to administer.
- Questions examine food intake, weight loss, body mass index, psychological stress/acute disease incidence, neuropsychological problems, and mobility.[7]

Instant Nutritional Assessment
- A simple and practical nutrition-screening tool.
- Combines three elements: lymphocyte count, albumin, and weight change.
- High degree of accuracy when three elements combined.[4]

Nutritional screening initiative and the DETERMINE Checklist
- Self-administered screening tool.
- Includes 10 questions about risk factors for malnutrition.
- Total scores of 6 or higher (highest score is 21) indicate a need for further assessment.[10]

Malnutrition Risk Scale (SCALES)
- Outpatient screening tool for malnutrition.
- The acronym SCALES represents the five elements of the tool: sadness, cholesterol, and loss of weight, eating problems, and shopping.
- A score of three or higher suggests high risk for malnutrition.[11]

Malnutrition Screening Tool
- A quick, valid, and reliable two-item tool.[12]
- The tool asks about unplanned weight loss and poor appetite.
- If the patient reports weight loss or poor appetite, he or she may be at risk for malnutrition.

Food Expectations, Long Term Care
- A 28-item, four-domain instrument developed to measure nursing home resident food satisfaction.[13,14]
- Self-administered or administered by an evaluator who reads each item and marks the resident's response.

Box 4
Anthropometric and body composition measures

Serial body weight

Serial body weight is a useful way to identify a change in overall nutritional status.[7]

Body mass index

Body mass index (BMI) is used to determine body fat levels, with a BMI <18.5 kg/m² indicating underweight and an increased risk of mortality.[7] In older adults, BMI may be problematic, in that height measurement may be inaccurate secondary to physical changes related to aging. Thus, BMI may not accurately predict body composition in older adults.

Triceps skinfold

Triceps skinfold (TSF) is reflective of fat stores. It is measured using a skinfold caliper by measuring the mid-point between the acromion process and the alecranon process of the upper arm. An average of three measurements is used. Nutritional depletion is defined as a skinfold measure of <11.3 mm in women and <4.3 mm in men.[15]

Mid-upper arm circumference

Mid-upper arm circumference (MUAC) is a predictor of mortality in older adults living in nursing homes.[16] To determine MUAC, the mid-point of the upper arm is measured with a tape measure placed snugly against the skin. Once the TSF and MUAC are measured, a mid-arm muscle circumference (MAMC), an indicator of lean mass, can be calculated using the following equation MAMC = AC − (TSF × 0.314).[15] Older adults are considered nutritionally depleted when their measure falls below the tenth percentile, which is <17.2 cm in women and <19.6 cm in men.

Bioelectrical impedance analysis

Bioelectrical impedance analysis is an expensive, quick, and noninvasive tool used in clinical practice to estimate fat mass versus lean mass. The ideal percentage body fat for older adults is 27.6% to 34.4% for women and 20.3% to 26.7% for men.[7]

- Maintenance of good oral hygiene, sensible treatment of dysphagia and depression, and decreasing or limiting the number of prescribed and over-the-counter medications also play an important role in enhancing food intake.[2]
- Nutrients essential to older adults are protein and vitamin D. Deficiencies in these nutrients are associated with higher risk of falls.[18]

Box 5
Laboratory tests associated with poor nutrition

Serum albumin <3.5 g/dL

Serum prealbumin <11 mg/dL

Cholesterol <150 mg/dL

Leptin <4.0 μg/L in men, <6.48 μg/L in women

From Loreck E, Chimakurthi R, Steinle NI. Nutritional assessment of the geriatric patient: a comprehensive approach toward evaluating and managing nutrition. Clin Geriatr 2012;20(4):20–6.

- Older adults who reside in nursing homes are especially at risk for malnutrition. Improving the dining experience by offering food choice, select menus, and buffet dining have been successful in increasing food intake and decreasing weight loss.[19–21]
- Interdisciplinary referral to:
  - A speech-language pathologist to assess and treat dysphagia and swallowing problems.
  - A registered dietitian to assess and treat reversible nutritional issues or to develop a plan to initiate nutrition support.
  - A social worker to assist older adults and families to obtain access to home-delivered meals or other assistance programs.
  - A dentist for oral health issues.
  - A geriatric psychiatrist for mental health issues.
  - An occupational or physical therapist consultation for older adults with physical limitations.
  - A pharmacist to assist with nutrition-related medication management issues.[7]

DEHYDRATION

Dehydration is defined as a fluid imbalance caused by too little fluid intake or too much fluid lost, or both.[22] Dehydration can occur quickly in older adults and the effects are disastrous. With older age, the body struggles to maintain fluid balance secondary to changes in thirst response, total body fluid, and decline in kidney function.

The body's thirst response declines with age, thus the body may fail to signal for adequate fluid intake. Total body fluid also declines with age. After age 60 years, total body fluid decreases to 52% in men and 46% in women from previous adult averages of 60% in men and 52% in women.[23] Older age also leads to a decline in kidney function. This means that the kidneys are less able to concentrate urine, thus more water is lost in comparison with younger persons.[24]

Risk Factors

There are many factors associated with increased risk for dehydration in older adults (**Box 6**).[24–29]

Indicators of Hydration Status

When assessing hydration status, it is best to use a variety of evidence-based approaches to ensure reliability of findings. One such approach is the use of a urine color chart.[30,31] The eight-item urine color chart ranges from pale straw (number 1) to greenish brown (number 8).[30] Urine that is pale straw in color usually indicates normal hydration status. As urine darkens, hydration levels may be declining (after adjusting for changes secondary to foods or medications). A score of less than four on the urine color chart is preferred to indicate normal hydration.[24]

Serum markers also are used to evaluate hydration status. The most reliable laboratory measures of dehydration are serum sodium, serum osmolality, and the ratio of blood urea nitrogen to creatinine (**Box 7**). Unfortunately, laboratory tests only confirm or refute the diagnosis of dehydration; they are not preventative.[24]

Finally, an in-depth clinical assessment is equally important when assessing for dehydration. Physical symptoms of dehydration may include dry oral mucosa, decreased urine output, furrowed tongue, sunken eyes, decreased salivation, upper-body

---

Box 6
Dehydration risk factors in older adults

Age >85 years

Race; black people higher risk

Thirst reduction

Problems accessing water/fluids

Communication problems

Cognitive disorders (dementia, delirium)

Swallowing difficulties

Reduced appetite

Medications (eg, diuretics, laxatives, antipsychotics, anxiolytics)

Polypharmacy (prescribed more than four medications)

Acute pathology (eg, fever, vomiting, diarrhea)

Level of physical dependency

Environmental barriers

Lack of attention from caregivers

Concomitant conditions (frailty, diabetes, cancer, cardiac disease)

---

weakness, and rapid pulse.[32] The assessment of skin turgor at the sternum is the standard in younger adults; however, it is not a reliable indicator of dehydration in older adults because of normal skin elasticity changes attributed to aging.[32,33]

Nursing Implications

It is recommended that older adults with or without comorbidities should drink small amounts of water throughout the day. Consuming large amounts of fluid at any one time is not recommended.[24,34] The daily amount of fluid needed by most older adults is calculated using the following formula: 100 mL/kg for the first 10 kg of weight, 50 mL/kg for the next 10 kg of weight, and 15 mL/kg for the remaining weight.[35] Except for those elders needing to limit their fluid intake because of severe congestive heart failure or renal failure, older adults should strive to drink at least 1500 mL of fluid per day.[24] Specific approaches or steps to prevent dehydration are listed in **Box 8**.[24]

ELECTROLYTE IMBALANCE

As with other organs of the body, degenerative changes in the kidneys occur with aging. Around age 40 there is a gradual increase in cortical glomerulosclerosis and a

---

Box 7
Laboratory markers of dehydration

- Serum sodium levels >150 mEq/L
- Serum osmolality levels >300 mmol/kg
- Blood urea nitrogen/creatinine ratio of $\geq$25:1 mg/dL

Box 8
Steps to prevent dehydration in older adults

- Provide and make accessible fluids that older adults like and enjoy drinking.
- Teach older adults to drink even if they are not thirsty.
- Identify at-risk older adults.
- Evaluate and reduce the number of prescribed medications.
- Identify and treat treatable causes of dehydration, such as diarrhea and vomiting.
- Measure fluid intake and urinary output.
- Provide appropriately sized cups and glasses for older adults to handle and straws if necessary.
- Advise caregivers to offer small amounts of fluid each time they enter the room.
- Instruct caregivers to encourage the older adult to drink 8 oz of fluids between and at each meal.
- During hot weather, be especially vigilant to signs and symptoms of dehydration.
- Provide positive feedback to caregivers who provide fluids.

---

decline in renal plasma flow and the glomerular filtration rate. "These changes may be associated with an inability to excrete a concentrated or a dilute urine, ammonium, sodium, or potassium. Hypernatremia and hyponatremia are the most common electrolyte abnormalities found in the elderly and both are associated with a high mortality."[36(p308)]

Risk factors for electrolyte imbalance include greater than 80 years of age, female, reside in a nursing home, underlying infection, and a dementia diagnosis.[36] Contributing factors that could lead to developing hypernatremia in older adults are listed in **Box 9**.[36]

Medications also are known to cause electrolyte imbalance, specifically hyponatremia. In a 2014 class-by-class review of the literature,[37] antidepressant-induced hyponatremia was found to increase with the use of selective serotonin reuptake inhibitors and/or serotonin-norepinephrine reuptake inhibitors, such as venlafaxine (Effexor). This is of concern because hyponatremia is a risk factor for osteoporosis and bone fracture.[38]

Hyponatremia contributes to falls and fractures in two ways. First, it can result in mild cognitive impairment leading to unsteady gait and falls. Second, hyponatremia induces increased bone resorption contributing to osteoporosis and increased bone fragility.[39] Older adults who have experienced a fall with or without fracture should have a serum sodium checked and hyponatremia corrected, if present.[39]

Box 9
Contributing factors of hypernatremia

- An inability to obtain or get to water
- An increase in insensible loss of water secondary to fever
- A decline in urinary concentrating capacity leading to an inability to retain free water
- A decline in thirst

Hyperkalemia is another common electrolyte imbalance in older adults. Risk factors for hyperkalemia are listed in **Box 10**.[40]

Hyperkalemia is classified as either significant (serum potassium value >6.0 mEq/L), or moderate (5.0–6.0 mEq/L). Hyperkalemia is most commonly caused by either a high intake of potassium (supplements or potassium rich foods) or by extracellular redistribution of potassium from intracellular locations. Clinical symptoms of hyperkalemia are rare with values less than 6.0 mEq/L.[41]

Common symptoms of hyperkalemia include muscle weakness and electrocardiogram (ECG) changes, with the latter having the potential to progress to a life-threatening arrhythmia.[41] Significant hyperkalemia represents a medical emergency and requires immediate hospitalization.

The treatment of hyperkalemia includes treating the underlying comorbid diseases, decreasing or changing medications that are known to induce hyperkalemia, serial ECG monitoring, and a 24-hour urine to measure potassium excretion (to distinguish renal from extrarenal causes). Initial testing should include a basic metabolic panel, serum calcium, complete blood count, and an ECG.[41]

Hypokalemia is a serum potassium level less than 3.5 mEq/L. Moderate hypokalemia is serum potassium 2.5 to 3.0 mEq/L and severe less than 2.5 mEq/L. As with hyperkalemia, hypokalemia can manifest itself as muscle weakness and ECG changes. Hypokalemia is most commonly caused by urinary or gastrointestinal losses. Clinical symptoms typically do not show themselves until the serum potassium is less than 3.0 mEq/L.[42] The treatment of hypokalemia is typically potassium replacement or supplementation.

ORAL HEALTH

As the older adult population increases, oral health is becoming more important in the quest to maintain quality of life. Poor oral health can have a negative impact on overall quality of life secondary to tooth loss, pain, and discomfort and may prevent some older adults from chewing food properly. Poor oral health also can lead to poor nutrition.[43]

Xerostomia, or dry mouth, is one of the most common problems that negatively impacts food intake in older adults. Persons with xerostomia have difficulty in forming a food bolus or swallowing, and have a decreased ability to taste food. Xerostomia can lead to mucositis, dental caries, cracked lips, and fissured tongue.[44]

Box 10
Risk factors for hyperkalemia

- Length of hospital stay
- Use of the following medications
  - Nonsteroidal-anti inflammatory drugs
  - Spironolactone, a potassium-sparing diuretic
  - Angiotensin-converting enzyme inhibitors
  - Angiotensin receptor blockers
  - Heparin
- Two or more comorbid diseases
- Female gender
- History of renal injury

Box 11
Prevention of dental caries

- Adoption of good oral hygiene includes the use of
  - Rotating/oscillating toothbrushes
  - Topical fluoride
  - Daily mouth rinses
  - High fluoride toothpaste
  - Regular fluoride varnish application

Symptoms of xerostomia are temporary (short-term drug therapy, dehydration, anxiety) or long-standing. Causes of long-standing xerostomia include diseases of the salivary glands (ie, Sjögren syndrome, hepatitis C, and diabetes) and iatrogenic causes (drugs, local radiation, chemotherapy).[45,46] Xerostomia is most likely drug-induced in the older adult population and the risk increases with greater numbers of drugs taken.[45]

Older adults are at increased risk for dental caries secondary to increased gingival gum recession that exposes root surfaces and xerostomia. About 50% of persons age 75 years or older have dental caries affecting at least one tooth.[47–49] Prevention includes the adoption of good oral hygiene and a well-balanced diet. Examples of good oral hygiene are listed in **Box 11**.[47–49]

Older adults with cognitive impairment (mid-late stage dementia) are at increased risk for dental caries, periodontal disease, and oral infections.[50] In elders with prosthetic devices, such as dentures, the devices should be removed, inspected, and cleaned before bed and returned to the mouth in the morning.[50] Educating the caregiver on ways to prevent dental caries and periodontal disease is an important activity to enhance the older adult's oral health.

An older adult's functional abilities undoubtedly decline over time secondary to older age and debilitating diseases, such as osteoarthritis and/or rheumatoid arthritis. Modifications of toothbrush handles with Velcro or handlebar grips may help to enhance an elder's functional ability. Other approaches include the use of an electronic toothbrush with a wide, graspable handle or floss holders to help clean between teeth. Frequent dental cleanings and examinations can help promote optimal oral health in at-risk older adults.[50]

SUMMARY

Malnutrition, dehydration, electrolyte imbalance, and oral health in older adults are multifaceted and complex issues. No single tool, clinical marker, or approach accurately predicts nutritional status. However, integrating validated nutrition screening tools with anthropometric and laboratory data, the geriatric nurse or provider can get a more accurate picture of the older adult's nutrition status. When reversible causes of malnutrition are identified, evidence-based approaches should be undertaken, which may require referral to other disciplines.

REFERENCES

1. Morley JE. Pathophysiology of the anorexia of aging. Curr Opin Clin Nutr Metab Care 2013;1:27–32.

2. Morley JE. Undernutrition: a major problem in nursing homes. J Am Med Dir Assoc 2011;12:243–6.

3. Hickson M. Malnutrition and ageing. Postgrad Med J 2006;82:2–8.

4. Hajjar RR, Kamel HK, Denson K. Malnutrition in aging. Internet J Geriatr Gerontol 2004;1(1):1–16.

5. Omran ML, Morely JE. Assessment of protein energy malnutrition in older persons. Part 1: history, examination, body composition, and screening tools. Nutrition 2000;16:50–63.

6. Cruz-Jentoft AJ, Baeyens JP, Bauer JM, et al, European Working Group on Sarcopenia in Older People. Sarcopenia: European consensus on definition and diagnosis: report of the European Working Group on Sarcopenia. Age Ageing 2010;39(4):412–23.

7. Loreck E, Chimakurthi R, Steinle NI. Nutritional assessment of the geriatric patient: a comprehensive approach toward evaluating and managing nutrition. Clin Geriatr 2012;20(4):20–6.

8. Bourdel-Marchasson I. How to improve nutritional support in geriatric institutions. J Am Med Dir Assoc 2010;11:13–20.

9. Bauer JM, Kaiser MJ, Sieber CC. Evaluation of nutritional status in older persons: nutritional screening and assessment. Curr Opin Clin Nutr Metab Care 2010; 13(1):8–13.

10. Detsky AS, Baker JP, Mandelson RA, et al. Evaluating the accuracy of nutritional assessment techniques applied to hospitalized patients: methodology and comparisons. JPEN J Parenter Enteral Nutr 1984;8:153–9.

11. Morley JE. Death by starvation: a modern American problem? J Am Geriatr Soc 1989;37:184.

12. Ferguson M, Capra S, Bauer J, et al. Development of a valid and reliable malnutrition screening tool for adult acute hospital patients. Nutrition 1999;15(6): 458–64.

13. Crogan NL, Evans B, Velasquez D. Measuring nursing home resident satisfaction with food and food service: Initial testing of the FoodEx-LTC. J Gerontol A Biol Sci Med Sci 2004;59A(4):370–7.

14. Crogan NL, Evans B. The shortened food expectations: long-term care questionnaire: assessing nursing home residents' satisfaction with food and food service. J Gerontol Nurs 2006;32(11):50–9.

15. Burr ML, Phillips KM. Anthropometric norms in the elderly. Br J Nutr 1984;51(2): 165–9.

16. Allard JP, Aghdassi E, McArthur M, et al. Nutrition risk factors for the survival in elderly living in Canadian long-term care facilities. J Am Geriatr Soc 2004; 52(1):59–65.

17. Thompson FE, Subar AF. Dietary assessment methodology. 2012. Available at: http://www.indiana.gov/isdh/files/4_TAB__3.pdf. Accessed May 20, 2017.

18. Zoltick ES, Sahni S, McLean RR, et al. Dietary protein intake and subsequent falls in older men and women: the Framingham study. J Nutr Health Aging 2011;15(2): 147–52.

19. Calkins M, Brush J. Honoring individual choice in long-term residential communities when it involves risk: a person-centered approach. J Gerontol Nurs 2016; 42(8):12–7.

20. Crogan NL, Dupler AE, Short R, et al. Food choice can improve nursing home resident meal service and nutritional status. J Gerontol Nurs 2013;39(5):38–45.

21. Heaton G, Crogan NL, Short R, et al. Resident food choice: evolution of the facility menu using rate the food. Dietary Manager 2011;20:30–4.

22. Weinberg AD, Minaker KL. Dehydration. Evaluation and management in older adults. Council on Scientific Affairs, American Medical Association. JAMA 1995;274(1):1552–6.
23. Metheny NM. Fluid and electrolyte balance: nursing considerations. 4th edition. Philadelphia: Lippincott; 2000.
24. Mentes J. Oral hydration in older adults. Am J Nurs 2006;106(6):40–9.
25. Lavizzo-Mourey R, Johnson J, Stolley P. Risk factors for dehydration among elderly nursing home residents. J Am Geriatr Soc 1988;36(3):213–8.
26. Ciccone A, Allegra JR, Cochrane DG, et al. Age-related differences in diagnoses within the elderly population. Am J Emerg Med 1998;16(1):43–8.
27. Lancaster KJ, Smiciklas-Wright H, Heller DA, et al. Dehydration in black and white older adults using diuretics. Ann Epidemiol 2003;13(7):525–9.
28. Gaspar PM. Water intake of nursing home residents. J Gerontol Nurs 1999;25(4): 23–9.
29. Mezey M, Maslow K. Try this: recognition of dementia in hospitalized older adults. New York: Hartford Institute for Geriatric Nursing; 2004.
30. Armstrong LE, Maresh CM, Castellani JW, et al. Urinary indices of hydration status. Int J Sport Nutr 1994;4(3):265–79.
31. Mentes JC, Wakefield B, Culp K. Use of a color chart to monitor hydration status in nursing home residents. Biological Research for Nursing 2006;7(3):197–203.
32. Gross CR, Lindquist RD, Woolley AC, et al. Clinical indicators of dehydration severity in elderly patients. J Emerg Med 1992;10(3):267–74.
33. Eaton D, Bannister P, Mulley GP, et al. Axillary sweating in clinical assessment of dehydration in ill elderly patients. BMJ 1994;308(6939):1271.
34. Luckey AE, Parsa CJ. Fluid and electrolytes in the aged. Arch Surg 2003;138(10): 1055–60.
35. Chidester JC, Spanger AA. Fluid intake in the institutionalized elderly. J Am Diet Assoc 1997;97(1):23–8.
36. Schlanger LE, Bailey JL, Sands JM. Electrolytes in the aging. Adv Chronic Kidney Dis 2010;17(4):308–19.
37. De Picker L, Van Den Eede F, Dumont G, et al. Antidepressants and the risk of hyponatremia: a class-by-class review of literature. Psychosomatics 2014;55(6): 536–47.
38. Amar AO, Holm JP, Jensen JE. Hyponatremia is a risk factor for osteoporosis and bone fracture. Ugeskr Laeger 2016;178(37) [pii: V03160210].
39. Negri AL, Ayus JC. Hyponatremia and bone disease. Rev Endocr Metab Disord 2016;18(1):67–78.
40. Turgutalp K, Bardak S, Helvaci I, et al. Community-acquired hyperkalemia in elderly patients: risk factors and clinical outcomes. Ren Fail 2016;38(9):1405–12.
41. Yarlagadda SG, Suneja M, Thuraisingham R. Hyperkalemia evaluation. Epocrates. Available at: www.epocrates.com. Accessed October 15, 2016.
42. Kabadi U, Suneja M, Hathiwala SC, et al. Hypokalemia evaluation. Epocrates. Available at: www.epocrates.com. Accessed October 15, 2016.
43. Eke PI, Wei L, Borgnakke WS, et al. Periodontitis prevalence in adults >65 years of age, in the USA. Periodontol 2000 2016;72(1):76–95.
44. Stein P, Aalboe J. Dental care in the frail older adult: special considerations and recommendations. J Calif Dent Assoc 2015;43(7):363–8.
45. Glore RJ, Spiteri-Staines K, Paleri V. A patient with dry mouth. Clin Otolaryngol 2009;34:358–63.
46. Porter SR, Scully C, Hegarty AM. An update of the etiology and management of xerostomia. Oral Surg Oral Med Oral Pathol 2004;97(1):28–46.

47. Centers for Disease Control and Prevention (CDC). Public health and aging: retention of natural teeth among older adults—United States, 2002. MMWR Morb Mortal Wkly Rep 2003;52(50):1226–9.

48. U.S. Department of Health and Human Services. Oral health in America: a report of the Surgeon general. Rockville (MD): U.S. Department of Health and Human Services, National Institute of Dental and Craniofacial Research, National Institute of Health; 2000.

49. Gregory D, Hyde S. Root caries in older adults. J Calif Dent Assoc 2015;43(8): 439–45.

50. Yellowitz JA. Geriatric health and functional issues. In: Patton LL, Glick M, editors. The ADA practical guide to patients with medical conditions. 2nd edition. Hoboken (NJ): John Wiley & Sons, Inc.; 2016. p. 405–22.

Geriatric Urinary Incontinence

Jessica A.R. Searcy, DNP, FNP-BC, WHNP-BC

KEYWORDS

- Geriatric • Women • Aging • Urinary incontinence • Mixed incontinence
- Stress incontinence • Urge urinary incontinence • Management

KEY POINTS

- Urinary incontinence (UI) is a prevalent problem for all people internationally, peaking in the geriatric population.
- UI is often classified as the context in which urine is involuntary lost and can be correlated with other urinary, bowel, or pelvic symptoms.
- UI screening should be implemented across all stages of health care in an effort to identify those who suffer in silence with UI symptoms.
- A thorough history, comprehensive examination, and thorough analysis of other diagnostic tools can help identify the type of UI with which the patient suffers.
- Once the type of UI has been identified, conservative measures, such as pelvic floor muscle training or bladder training, may be implemented along with lifestyle modifications. Various medications and other electronic forms of treatment are available to help decrease symptoms of UI.

INTRODUCTION

Urinary incontinence (UI), or involuntary urine loss, is a lower urinary tract symptom resulting from impaired bladder storage.[1,2] UI can result from a variety of causes ranging from transient infections to structural abnormalities to pelvic floor dysfunction. UI persists as a significant disease of morbidity in the United States and worldwide affecting men and women across the lifespan with peak prevalence in the geriatric population. Though the extent of symptoms and impairment may vary, evidence continues to show the effects of UI on a woman's quality of life include limitations of physical activity and psychological burdens. This article provides a general review of current evidence on nontransient presentations of UI, including stress, urge, and mixed incontinence, and implications for health care providers caring for geriatric women with UI.

Disclosure Statement: As the author of this article, I have no affiliations or disclosures nor have I received financial compensation for the work associated with this article.
Women's Health Nurse Practitioner Program, Vanderbilt University School of Nursing, 461 21st Avenue South, Nashville, TN 37240, USA
E-mail address: Jessica.searcy@vanderbilt.edu

Nurs Clin N Am 52 (2017) 447–455
http://dx.doi.org/10.1016/j.cnur.2017.04.002

OVERVIEW

UI is often concurrent with aging of the lower urinary tract, infections of the urinary tract, and also non-genitourinary causes including chronic conditions such as diabetes mellitus, cognitive impairment, neurological conditions, and obesity, and is not considered normal in the aging process.[2–7] Continence requires optimal cognitive functioning, appropriate structure and functioning (contracting and relaxing) of the detrusor muscle and urethra, appropriate support of the pelvic floor from muscles (levator ani complex) and connective tissue, and appropriate innervation from the peripheral nervous system.[2,3,7–9] UI is the one of the most common pelvic floor disorders resulting from pelvic floor dysfunction and frequently occurs concomitantly with other pelvic floor disorders, such as fecal incontinence or pelvic organ prolapse.[10] Unintentional urinary leakage can occur when pressure inside the bladder increases above the pressure within the urethra.[2] Alteration of the pressures within the bladder and the urethra can occur from various underlying pathologic conditions.[2] The numerous risk factors for UI include age, childbearing, type of obstetric deliveries, obesity, diabetes, poor physical function, and poor cognitive function and memory loss.[3,4,6,11–13] If structural or neurologic abnormalities are present, individuals may experience a variety of other urinary storage or sensory symptoms, including frequency, urgency, and decreased bladder sensation.[1] Possible factors leading to UI include delirium, infection, atrophic urethritis and vaginitis, pharmaceuticals, psychological disorders, excessive urine output, restricted mobility, and stool impaction (DIAPPERS). These criteria are frequently used in evidence to highlight transient and reversible causes of UI,[3,14] all of which should be considered and ruled out when a geriatric patient presents with UI.

Specific to women, a lack of estrogen production from the ovaries characteristic of menopause can precipitate bladder symptoms such as UI.[15] This lack of estrogen to the female pelvis, formerly known as atrophic vaginitis or vulvovaginal atrophy, is known as Genitourinary Symptom of Menopause, and should be considered as a precipitating cause or influence of UI and is highlighted in the acronym DIAPPERS as a transient cause of UI.[3,15]

Specific types of UI are categorized based on symptoms.[1] Stress UI (SUI) occurs during a physical stressor and increase in intra-abdominal pressure (coughing, sneezing, laughing, or physical exertion) in which support or mechanical closure of the urethra is compromised, as with hypermobility of the urethra or intrinsic sphincter deficiency.[1,9,16–18] Urge UI (UUI) occurs along with a sudden, compelling urge to urinate and can be attributed to multiple causes of detrusor instability and overactivity.[1,9,17,18] Mixed UI (MUI) is the combination of SUI and UUI in which leakage occurs in the presence of a physical stressor and with an intense urge to void.[1,2,18,19] The SUI and UUI symptoms experienced with MUI are not required to occur at the same time; instead, the patient may experience episodes of isolated SUI and isolated UUI. SUI is commonly seen in younger and middle aged-women, and UUI and MUI is commonly seen in geriatric women.[18] Additional UI symptoms include postural incontinence, continuous incontinence, insensible incontinence, and coital incontinence.[1]

PREVALENCE

Prevalence rates for UI in the general population and across the world can vary based on cultural differences, types and frequency of symptoms, perceptions, reporting inconsistencies, and research-based differences.[3] True prevalence rates are most likely higher than what is recorded due to the underreporting of symptoms from patients and the underdiagnosing from providers.[19] The 5th International Consultation on Incontinence reported UI prevalence among population studies as 6% to 69% with most concluding that 25% to 45% of individuals suffer from UI symptoms.[3] An estimated 30% to 60% of middle-aged and geriatric women, and 2% to 34% of men, suffer episodes of UI.[3] UI rates in women are estimated to be twice as high as those in men, and UI rates vary between the genders based on the type of incontinence, age, and other factors.[3,5,20] Because UI can be concomitant with other diseases, including diabetes and overactive bladder, identifying prevalence of isolated UI is complex.[21]

Gender Prevalence

UI in women can occur at a young age, including nulliparous women and those younger than 18 years old.[22,23] Most UI cases are attributed to SUI, which is approximately 10% to 39% and up to greater than 50% of cases, depending on the source.[3] The second most common type of UI is MUI, at approximately 7.5% to 25% of cases.[3] UUI is the least common form but is more common in women than men and often associated with overactive bladder.[18,20] Isolated UUI accounts for 1% to 7% of leakage in women, and it can be found in the presence of other types of incontinence.[3] By 2050, the projected number of women who suffer with UI related to pelvic floor dysfunction is estimated to be approximately 28.4 million.[24]

Though male UI rates are less than half than of those of women, current evidence has found that 1% to 39% of men suffer from UI symptoms.[3] UUI is the most prevalent form in men, estimated to cause 40% to 80% of cases.[3] UUI is the primary cause of the higher rates of UI in elderly men.[3] MUI is attributed to 10% to 30% of cases, whereas SUI accounts for less than 10% of cases.[3]

Geriatric Prevalence

UI rates are influenced by situational factors. UI trends increase with age even though these symptoms are not considered to be a normal part of aging.[7,10,11,25] More than 50% of women and 25% of men aged 65 years and older, not residing health care facilities or institutions, reported symptoms of UI of varying severities.[5] Approximately 50% of geriatric men and women living in residential care facilities reported UI, and another 50% reported both fecal and UI.[5,26] Of men and women receiving home health care, 40% reported symptoms of UI.[5] Geriatric individuals in short-term and long-term nursing home care who were unable to maintain bladder control ranged from approximately 36% to 70%.[5] Rates of UI and pelvic floor disorders have risen throughout the years and are predicted to continue rising as the geriatric population in America continues to grow.[3,24] These statistics confirm that presence of UI affects aging women in all living situations. Caregivers, support staff, and health care providers at all levels of the health care system need to know how to care for those with UI.

BURDEN
Economic Burden

The economic burden of UI occurs on the level of the individual but also extends to the workforce and to national costs. Because UI often occurs concomitantly with other diseases, such as overactive bladder, the isolated cost of UI can be ambiguous.[21] Costs associated with UI can include direct costs (eg, health care provider visits, laboratory evaluation expenses, medications, procedures, therapies) and indirect costs (eg, lack of productivity or loss of time at work, costs for sanitary products and at-home supplies) are significant.[21,27] Though UI occurs in women and men, women suffer from the greatest individual costs associated with UI.[21] In a randomized control trial assessing UI costs, 94% of a cohort of 617 women used resources to manage UI symptoms, including incontinence, and greater than 50% of women had additional laundry because of their UI symptoms.[27] The annual mean cost of general UI care ranged from $751 to $1277 for all women with many of those willing to spend up more than $1400 annually to seek relief from symptoms.[27] UI symptoms can precipitate disability and absence from work but are not correlated with exiting the workforce.[28,29] Sung and colleagues[30] (2010) identified increasing trends of pelvic floor dysfunction, including UI. The direct costs for UI in the ambulatory care alone were $68.7 million in 2005 through 2006. The national and global economic burden of UI, including health care costs and visits, is predicted to increase as the population ages.[30–32]

Quality of Life and Psychological Burden

The cost of UI extends beyond monetary costs because decreased quality of life and psychological burdens often stem from symptoms. UI symptoms can cause instrumental impairment in activities of daily living and negative quality of life.[20,33] The psychological symptoms experienced by women are diverse and may include anxiety, depression, and embarrassment.[28,34,35] UI can also contribute to impaired sexual function.[36,37] The severity of these burdens can vary with category of UI from which the patient suffers and severity of symptoms.[20,33,34]

CLINICAL APPLICATION
Evidence-Based Guidelines

Current national and international guidelines help guide practitioners caring for geriatric patients with UI. Dowling-Castronovo and Bradway[38] (2012) updated their nursing protocol specific to geriatric UI management in the setting of acute care. The American Medical Directors Association updated their guideline on geriatric UI in the long-term setting in 2012.[39] The American College of Physicians developed a guideline in 2013 related to nonsurgical UI management for women.[19] The guidelines are available through the National Guideline Clearinghouse for provider reference. Other international guidelines, protocols, and recommendations on UI diagnosis and management are also available for reference.[3,13,26]

History

Proactive screening for UI by health care providers should implemented for geriatric women in all settings because women often do not disclose symptoms of UI to providers due to various factors, including embarrassment, not identifying symptoms as severe, established mechanisms of coping with symptoms, or misconception that UI is a normal process of aging.[19,26,40,41] Geriatric women in the all health care settings should be screened for UI symptoms.[26,38] Provider-driven questions asking about the presence or absence of unintended or accidental urine leakage and when it occurs can be sufficient for initial UI screening; however, the 5th International Consultation on Incontinence committee[3] recommends the use of standardized questions for initial UI assessment.[3,42,43]

If UI symptoms are identified, a detailed patient history from the patient or caregiver helps identify the type of UI, precipitating and influential factors, and identifies symptoms as acute or chronic.[1,3,8,19,26,33,38,44] A detailed history is especially imperative in geriatrics because UI can stem from urinary or nonurinary causes, and may present as transient or persistent symptoms.[45] Patient history should include onset, duration, frequency, severity, aggravating or alleviating factors, associated symptoms (urologic and nonurologic), and past or current treatments to help identify context of leakage, as well as symptoms that are most bothersome.[2,3,14,18,26,42,44,45] Other bladder dysfunction and pelvic dysfunction symptoms should be assessed, including dysuria, frequency, urgency, nocturia, hesitancy, pelvic pain, and vaginal dryness, to identify overall pelvic health of the patient.[1,26,42] Identifying a patient's medical history (ie, bowel, menstrual, obstetric, and sexual history), surgical history, and current medications and supplements provides a complete picture of the patient's overall health status, risk factors, and helps identify potential influencing factors on symptoms.[3,19,26,46]

Assessment

No current research exists addressing physical examination components in assessment of UI, but ruling out transient causes versus nontransient causes is the goal of the physical examination.[3,18,46] A focused physical examination, including neurologic, abdominal, genitourinary, pelvic, and rectal examinations, may unveil various contributing factors associated with UI symptoms, such as sensory impairment, neurologic function, cough, impaired mobility or muscle strength, bladder distention, genitourinary syndrome of menopause, pelvic organ prolapse, and compromised skin integrity.[3,7,8,13,26,44] A current body mass index measurement should be calculated.[3] Advanced assessments, including the cotton swab test, sitting and standing Valsalva, cough stress test assessing for SUI, pelvic organ prolapse assessment, and pelvic muscle strength, can help grade abnormal examination findings and identify additional physical findings potentially contributing to UI symptoms.[3,13,26,46,47]

Other sources of assessment information include frequency-volume charts, pad weights, and questionnaires. A frequency-volume chart, otherwise known as a voiding diary, is an essential part of the assessment process. It should be completed by patients over 3 24-hour periods to help to quantify time and volume of voids, UI episodes, perineal pad changes, and fluid intake.[1-3,8,26,46,47] Pad tests are another optional objective test.[26] Previously, pad counts were used to grade severity of UI symptoms in patients. Current recommendations include use of incontinence pad weighing to accurately quantify urine loss and severity of UI episodes instead of counting the numbers of pads used during the day.[1,3,48] The use of validated and standardized symptom and quality of life questionnaires, such as the 3 incontinence questions, is helpful in screening patients and in acquiring the initial UI history; they can help in the assessment in turn by providing information on the extent of the UI symptoms, which can help evaluate treatment efficacy.[3,26,46,47]

Additional diagnostic testing to aid in ruling out transient causes and identifying the cause of UI may include urinalysis, urine culture, postvoid residuals, urodynamic studies, cystoscopy, and other forms of bladder testing and imaging.[3,13,26,47] A screening urinalysis is considered as fundamental to an initial UI assessment, and diagnostic urine culture can help identify urinary tract infections as well as underlying any abnormalities such as hematuria, pyuria, and bacteruria.[3,8,18,26] Postvoid residuals are an appropriate assessment tool to investigate for incomplete bladder emptying in correlation with UI symptoms.[3,26,47] More invasive imaging and tests, such as urodynamics (eg, cystometry, uroflowmetry, and pressure flow studies), cystourethrography, cystourethroscopy, and pelvic ultrasound are potential diagnostic tools used in the outpatient urology and urogynecology clinical settings to narrow down underlying pathophysiology causing UI to more accurately direct care management.[8,13,18,26,45-47]

Clinical Management

Clinical management of UI depends on various factors, including UI classification, level of care, location of care, patient safety, patient preferences, and available resources. Management recommendations for SUI and UUI are pelvic floor muscle therapy

(PFMT) and bladder training, respectively. A combination of PFMT and bladder training is recommended for patients with MUI.[13,19,26,38] Multiple studies have shown PFMT as efficacious for alleviating UI symptoms.[19,49] PFMT and bladder training are considered as behavioral inventions, along with timed voiding, patient education, positive reinforcement, and lifestyle modifications that can be initiated by providers at any level of care.[14] Systemic pharmacotherapy is not recommended for SUI treatment.[19] Medications such as anticholinergics, including antimuscarinics, and beta-3 adrenergic agonists are recommended for UUI only if initial bladder training is ineffective in controlling symptoms and should be initiated and monitored with caution due to risk for side effects in the geriatric population.[13,18,19,26] Estrogen replacement's efficacy in alleviating UI symptoms remains controversial, lacking sufficient evidence at this time, and should not be recommended routinely for treatment of SUI.[13,19,26,45] Additional management options include pelvic floor electrical stimulation and vaginal cones or weights available at specialty level of care.[13,26] There are numerous surgical treatments for SUI and UUI available for patients when they are referred to a specialist, including in-office urethral bulking agents, surgical placement of urethral slings and bladder neck suspensions for SUI, and intradetrusor botulinum toxin injection therapy and sacral neuromodulation for patients with UUI associated with overactive bladder if conservative or pharmacologic therapies fail.[7,17,18,26,50–53] In 2013, the US Food and Drug Administration (FDA) approved detrusor botulinum toxin injections for UUI symptoms; these injections can be given in a specialty office and duration of treatment varies.[17] Sacral neuromodulation aims to simulate the sacral nerve root to control urination and can be office-based as with 12-week course of weekly percutaneous tibial nerve simulation in office, or through the surgical implantation of sacral neuromodulator system.[17,52] Surgical sacral neuromodulation includes implantation of the Medtronic Interstim Therapy device, currently FDA- approved for bladder dysfunction, including UI, and for fecal incontinence, and it has shown efficacy in decreasing symptoms of UI.[51,52]

The efficacy of lifestyle modifications is debated. For overweight and obese women, a 5% to 10% weight loss through exercise has shown to decrease UI symptoms.[32,54,55] Therefore, weight loss is recommended for women with body mass index higher than normal range,[18,19] and weight loss counseling and support should be initiated at all levels of care.[14] Overall, the short-term and long-term outcomes of other lifestyle modifications, such as reduction of caffeine and alcohol, smoking cessation, and physical activity level, need to be investigated.[56,57] Water and fluid restriction should not be recommended for the management of UI symptoms, and other management techniques, such as eliminating dietary bladder irritants and regulating bowel function, may help in alleviating symptoms.[14,26]

Additional management considerations for the geriatric patients include skin hygiene and breakdown prevention with proper cleansing of the urethral meatus, external genitalia, and perineum and elimination of wet undergarments and pads after UI episodes.[26,38] Clothing and environmental changes may need consideration to improve continence efforts, such as decreasing thickness or layering of clothing for easier removal, ensuring clear walk ways to the toilet, and having lighting and handrails around the toilet.[26]

SUMMARY

UI poses a significant problem among geriatric women and in women across the lifespan in all settings of health care. The significance of UI in the lives of patients and the health care system is projected to increase in the upcoming years. Nurses work at every level in the health care system and can, therefore, advocate for the health and wellness of women suffering with UI symptoms. Nurses should understand the extent of UI problems, potential resources for referral, and options for treatment. Nurses should implement proactive screening, thorough assessment, and accurate diagnosis to help enhance outcomes for these patients through holistic plans of care or referrals for specialty evaluation or treatment modalities.

REFERENCES

1. Haylen BT, Ridder D, Freeman RM, et al. An International Urogynecological Association (IUGA)/International Incontinence Society (ICS) joint report on the terminology for female pelvic floor dysfunction. Neurourol Urodyn 2010;29(1):4–20.
2. Sheng Y, Miller JM. Urinary incontinence. In: Schuiling KD, Likis FE, editors. Women's gynecologic health. 3rd edition. Burlington (MA): Jones and Bartlett Learning; 2017. p. 25–548.
3. Abrams P, Cardozo L, Khoury S, et al. Incontinence, 5th International Consultation on Incontinence. Paris, February, 2012. 2013. Available at: http://www.icud.info/PDFs/INCONTINENCE%202013.pdf. Accessed November 26, 2016.
4. Doshi AM, Van Den Eeden SK, Morrill MY, et al. Women with diabetes: understanding urinary incontinence and help seeking behavior. J Urol 2010;184(4): 1402–7.
5. Gorina Y, Schappert S, Bercovitz A, et al. Prevalence of incontinence among older Americans. National Center for Health Statistics. Vital Health Stat 2014; 3(36):1–33.
6. Lawrence JM, Lukacz ES, Liu IA, et al. Pelvic floor disorders, diabetes, and obesity in women. Diabetes Care 2007;30(10):2536–41.
7. Richman SM, Drickamer MA. Gynecologic care of elderly women. J Am Med Dir Assoc 2007;8(4):219–33.
8. McDonough RC, Ryan ST. Diagnosis and management of lower urinary tract dysfunction. Surg Clin North Am 2016;96(3):441–52.
9. Rahn DD, Roshanraven SM. Pathophysiology of urinary incontinence, voiding dysfunction, and overactive bladder. Obstet Gynecol Clin North Am 2009; 36(3):463–74.
10. Nygaard I, Barber MD, Burgio KL, et al. Prevalence of symptomatic pelvic floor disorders in US women. JAMA 2008;300(11):1311–6.
11. Kepenekci I, Keskinkilin B, Akinsu F. Prevalence of pelvic floor disorders in the female population and the impact of age, mode of delivery, and parity. Dis Colon Rectum 2011;54(1):85–94.
12. Tahtinen RM, Cartwright R, Tsui JF, et al. Long term impact of mode of delivery on stress urinary incontinence and urgency urinary incontinence: a systematic review and meta-analysis. Eur Urol 2016;70(1):148–58.
13. Thüroff JW, Abrams P, Andersson K, et al. EAU guidelines on urinary incontinence. Eur Urol 2011;59(3):387–400.
14. Newman DK, Wein AJ. Office-based behavioral therapy for management of incontinence and other pelvic disorders. Urol Clin North Am 2013;40(4):613–35.
15. Ward K, Deneris A. Genitourinary syndrome of menopause: a new name for an old condition. Nurse Pract 2016;41(7):29–33.
16. Aleksic I, De EJ. Surgical management of female voiding dysfunction. Surg Clin North Am 2016;96(3):469–90.
17. MacLachlan LS, Rovner ES. New treatments for incontinence. Adv Chronic Kidney Dis 2015;22(4):279–88.
18. Deng DY. Urinary incontinence in women. Med Clin North Am 2011;95(1):101–9.

19. Qaseem A, Dallas P, Forclea MA, et al. Clinical guidelines committee of the American College of Physicians. Nonsurgical management of urinary incontinence in women: a clinical practice guideline from the American College of Physicians. Ann Intern Med 2014;161(6):429–40.

20. Sims J, Browning C, Lundgren-Lindquist B, et al. Urinary incontinence in a community sample of older adults: prevalence and impact on quality of life. Disabil Rehabil 2011;33(15–16):1389–98.

21. Ganz ML, Smalarz AM, Krupski TL, et al. Economic costs of overactive bladder in the United States. Urology 2010;75(3):526–32, 532.e1-18.

22. Ng SF, Lok MK, Pang SM, et al. Stress urinary incontinence in younger women in primary care: prevalence and opportunistic intervention. J Womens Health (Larchmt) 2014;23(1):65–8.

23. O'Halloran T, Bell RJ, Robinson PJ, et al. Urinary incontinence in young nulligravid women: a cross-sectional analysis. Ann Intern Med 2012;157(2):87–93.

24. Wu JM, Hundley AF, Fulton RG, et al. Forecasting the prevalence of pelvic floor disorders in U.S. women 2010-2050. Obstet Gynecol 2009;114(6):1278–83.

25. Lawrence JM, Lukacz ES, Mager CW, et al. Prevalence and co-occurrence of pelvic floor disorders in community-dwelling women. Obstet Gynecol 2008;111(3): 678–85.

26. Nishizawa O, Ishizuka O, Okamura K, et al. Guidelines for management of urinary incontinence. Int J Urol 2008;15(10):857–74.

27. Subak LL, Brubaker L, Chai TC, et al. High costs of urinary incontinence among women electing surgery to treat stress incontinence. Obstet Gynecol 2008; 111(4):899–907.

28. Hung KJ, Awtrey CS, Tsai AC. Urinary incontinence, depression, and economic outcomes in a cohort of women between ages of 54 and 65 years. Obstet Gynecol 2014;123(4):822–7.

29. Kleinman NL, Chen CI, Atkinson A, et al. Economic burden of urge urinary incontinence in the workplace. J Occup Environ Med 2014;56(3):266–9.

30. Sung VW, Washington B, Raker CA. Costs of ambulatory care related to female pelvic floor disorders in the United States. Am J Obstet Gynecol 2010;202(5): 483.e1-e4.

31. Milsom I, Coyne KS, Nicholson S, et al. Global prevalence and economic burden of urgency urinary incontinence: a systematic review. Eur Urol 2014;65(1):79–95.

32. Subak LL, Richter HE, Hunskaar S. Obesity and urinary incontinence: Epidemiology and clinical research update. J Urol 2009;182(6 Suppl):S2–7.

33. Frick AC, Huang AJ, Van Den Eden SK, et al. Mixed urinary incontinence: greater impact on quality of life. J Urol 2009;182(2):596–600.

34. Coyne KS, Kvasz M, Ireland AM, et al. Urinary incontinence and its relationship to mental health and health- related quality outcomes of life in men and women in Sweden, United Kingdom, and the United States. Eur Urol 2012;61(1):88–95.

35. Melville JL, Delaney K, Newton K, et al. Incontinence severity and major depression in incontinent women. Obstet Gynecol 2005;106(3):585–92.

36. Lim R, Liong ML, Leong WS, et al. Effect of stress urinary incontinence on the sexual function of couples and quality of life of patients. J Urol 2016;196(1):153–8.

37. Su CC, Sun BY, Jiann BP. Association of urinary incontinence and sexual function in women. Int J Urol 2015;22(1):109–13.

38. Dowling-Castronovo A, Bradway C. Urinary incontinence. In: Boltz M, Capezuti E, Fulmer T, et al, editors. Evidence-based geriatric nursing protocols for best practice. 4th edition. New York: Springer Publishing Company; 2012. p. 363–87.

39. National Guideline Clearinghouse (NGC). Guideline summary: Urinary incontinence in the long term care setting. In: National Guideline Clearinghouse (NGC) [Web site]. Rockville (MD): Agency for Healthcare Research and Quality (AHRQ); 2012. Available: https://guideline.gov. Accessed May 24, 2017.
40. Cameron AP, Heidelbaugh JJ, Jimbo M. Diagnosis and office based treatment of urinary incontinence in adults. Part one: diagnosis and testing. Ther Adv Urol 2013;5(4):181–7.
41. Visser E, De Bock GH, Boudewijn JK, et al. Systematic screening for urinary incontinence in older women: who could benefit from it? Scand J Prim Health Care 2012;30(1):21–8.
42. Bickley LS, Szilagyi PG, editors. Bates' guide to physical examination and history taking. 11th edition. Philadelphia: Wolters Kluwer Health/Lippincott Williams & Wilkins; 2013.
43. Visser E, Dekker JH, Verneulen KM, et al. The effect of systematic screening of older women for urinary incontinence on treatment uptake: the URINO trial. Maturitas 2013;74(4):334–40.
44. Testa A. Understanding urinary incontinence in adults. Urol Nurs 2015;35(2):82–6.
45. DeMaagd GA, Davenport TC. Management of urinary incontinence. P T 2012;37(6):345–61. Available at: https://www.ncbi.nlm.nih.gov/pmc/articles/PMC3411204/pdf/ptj3706345.pdf.
46. Khandelwal C, Kistler C. Diagnosis of urinary incontinence. Am Fam Physician 2013;87(8):543–50. Available at: http://www.aafp.org/afp/2013/0415/p543.pdf.
47. Wieslander CK. Clinical approach and office evaluation of the patient with pelvic floor dysfunction. Obstet Gynecol Clin North Am 2009;36(3):445–62.
48. Tsui JF, Shah MB, Weinberger JM, et al. Pad count is a poor measure of the severity of urinary incontinence. J Urol 2013;190(5):1787–90.
49. Dumoulin C, Hay-Smith EJ, Mac Habée-Séguin G. Pelvic floor muscle training versus no treatment, or inactive control treatments, for urinary incontinence in women. Cochrane Database Syst Rev 2014;(5):CD005654.
50. Amundsen CL, Richter HE, Menefee S, et al. The refractory overactive bladder: sacral neuromodulation vs. Botulinum toxin assessment: ROSETTA trial. Contemp Clin Trials 2014;37(2):272–83.
51. Fulton M, Peters KM. Neuromodulation for voiding dysfunction and fecal incontinence: a urology perspective. Urol Clin North Am 2012;39(3):405–12.
52. Kacker R, Lay A, Das A. Electrical and mechanical office-based neuromodulation. Urol Clin North Am 2013;40(4):581–9.
53. Smaldone MC, Ristau BT, Leng WW. Botulinum toxin therapy for neurogenic detrusor overactivity. Urol Clin North Am 2010;37(4):567–80.
54. Subak LL, Whitcomb E, Shen H, et al. Weight loss: a novel and effective treatment for urinary incontinence. J Urol 2005;174(1):190–5.
55. Wing RR, West DS, Grady D, et al. Effect of weight loss on urinary incontinence in overweight and obese women: results at 12 and 18 months. J Urol 2010;184(3):1005–10.
56. Imamura M, Williams K, Wells M, et al. Lifestyle interventions for the treatment of urinary incontinence in adults [review]. Cochrane Database Syst Rev 2015;(12):CD003505.
57. Jura YH, Townsend MK, Curhan GC, et al. Caffeine intake, and the risk of stress, urgency, and mixed urinary incontinence. J Urol 2011;185(5):1775–80.

Polypharmacy and Medication Management in Older Adults

Jennifer Kim, DNP, GNP-BC, FNAP*,
Abby Luck Parish, DNP, ANP-BC, GNP-BC, FNAP

KEYWORDS

- Polypharmacy • Elderly • Adverse drug event • Potentially inappropriate medication

KEY POINTS

- Polypharmacy is a common clinical issue in older adults; approximately 30% of senior citizens take at least 5 or more medications.
- The normal changes of aging and physical changes associated with disease predispose older adults to an increased sensitivity to prescription and over-the-counter medications.
- Nurses should refer to the Beers Criteria and screening tool of older people's prescriptions (STOPP) criteria when questioning the appropriateness of an elderly patient's medications.
- In lieu of pharmacologic measures, nurses should use patient-centered, evidence-based nonpharmacologic strategies to treat common symptoms.

THE PROBLEM OF POLYPHARMACY IN OLDER ADULTS
Background and Significance

Although prescribed and over-the-counter medications may improve a wide range of health problems, they also may cause or contribute to harm, especially in older adults. Current-day medication regimens for chronic health conditions are often complex, and such complexity has the potential for negative consequences. Older adults are disproportionately affected, as they typically have more disease conditions for which medication regimens are prescribed. Polypharmacy in older adults is a global problem that has recently worsened. Approximately 30% of adults age 65 and older in developed countries take 5 or more medications.[1] Although older adults make up approximately 14.5% of the US population, elderly individuals purchase 33% of all prescription drugs, and this proportion is expected to increase to 50% by the year 2040.[2,3] Prevention and management of medical conditions typically requires the

Disclosure Statement: Authors have nothing to disclose.
Vanderbilt University School of Nursing, 461 21st Avenue South, Nashville, TN 37240, USA
* Corresponding author.
E-mail address: jennifer.kim@vanderbilt.edu

use of medications, and medical management regimens have become increasingly complex. Polypharmacy may be the unintended consequence of the increasing use of clinical practice guidelines.

Polypharmacy is a common clinical issue in older adults. It not only includes pre-scribed medications but also over-the-counter and herbal preparations. Polyphar-macy is most commonly defined in the health care literature as taking 5 or more medications. Hyperpolypharmacy has been described as taking 10 or more medica-tions.[4] Polypharmacy in the older adult population is not surprising, as this population has a high prevalence of medical comorbidities. Nurses who work in all health care settings (hospital, ambulatory care, nursing home) are regularly confronted with the problems associated with polypharmacy. Nursing home residents typically take the highest number of medications, with an average of 7 to 8 different medications per month.[5,6] Forty percent of residents take more than 9 medications.[6]

The clinical consequences of polypharmacy in older adults have been well docu-mented. Polypharmacy is associated with the development and worsening of geriatric syndromes, including cognitive impairment, delirium, falls, frailty, urinary incontinence, and weight loss.[7] Polypharmacy in older adults also increases the risk of adverse drug events (ADEs) and avoidable hospitalizations. Polypharmacy also has financial conse-quences, as it results in increased health care costs for the patient and for the health care system. Treatment for medication errors and ADEs in the older adult population is estimated to cost more than 880 million dollars per year.[8] In 2012, inappropriate poly-pharmacy cost 1.3 billion dollars in avoidable health care costs.[9]

Causes of Polypharmacy

Although the etiology of polypharmacy may be either unknown or multifactorial, it is sometimes considered a proxy indicator for inappropriate medication use.[10] Prescrib-ing medications for frail older adults can be challenging, given their many medical, so-cial, and cognitive complexities. Although polypharmacy may be unavoidable in older adults who are being appropriately treated for multiple medical problems, it may also be inappropriate, with numerous risk factors placing older adults at high risk for its occurrence, including prescribing cascades and uncoordinated care.

Prescribing cascade
A prescribing cascade begins when a side effect or adverse drug reaction of a medica-tion is misinterpreted as a new health condition, thus resulting in the prescription of a new medication.[11] This new medication may lead to further side effects and subsequent medications and therapies to treat them. For example, an older adult taking a nonste-roidal anti-inflammatory drug (NSAID) for arthritic pain may develop hypertension, for which an antihypertensive medication is prescribed. An antihypertensive medication may cause dizziness, for which an antiemetic is prescribed. See **Table 1** for examples of common prescribing cascades.

Prescribing cascades are preventable causes of polypharmacy. Medications should be started at low doses, and the nurse should monitor patients for adverse reactions. The nurse should also promote the use of nonpharmacologic interventions to mitigate side effects. Finally, the nurse should assist the health care team by doing a thorough assessment of a patient's medication regimen, including start dates of all medications.

Uncoordinated care
Half of all people age 65 and older have at least 3 medical diagnoses, and one-fifth have 5 or more medical conditions.[16] It is not uncommon for older adults with multiple medical problems to be treated by different medical specialists. It is also not

Table 1		
Common prescribing cascades		
Initial Medication Prescribed	Side Effect	Secondary Medication Prescribed For Side Effect
Antipsychotic[11]	Extrapyramidal adverse effects	Levodopa, anticholinergics
Antiepileptic[12]	Nausea	Metoclopramide, domperidone
Antihypertensive[13]	Dizziness	Prochlorperazine
Cholinesterase inhibitor[14,15]	Incontinence	Anticholinergics (eg, oxybutynin)
NSAID[11]	Hypertension	Antihypertensive
Thiazide diuretic[11]	Hyperuricemia, gout	Allopurinol or colchicine

Data from Refs.[11–14]

uncommon for senior citizens to fill medications at different pharmacies. A lack of communication and collaboration between medical providers and between pharmacies may lead to duplication of therapy or the concurrent use of medications with drug interactions. This is also a potential problem when there is a lack of coordinated care when patients transition between different levels of care (eg, hospital, post–acute care, and home).

Pharmacokinetics and Aging

Pharmacokinetics is the study of the absorption, distribution, metabolism, and elimination of medications. The pharmacokinetics of medications in older adults is influenced by normal changes of aging and by physical changes associated with disease(s). Given these changes, older adults are more sensitive to many medications and are also more sensitive to medication changes. The bedside nurse should anticipate that older adult patients have the potential to respond differently to medications than other age groups.

Absorption

Reduced gastrointestinal motility and blood flow are associated with aging. There is also a reduction in gastric acid secretion, elevating gastric pH level. Although reduced gastrointestinal motility may result in an increased absorption rate of a medication, reduced gastric blood flow and an elevated gastric pH level may cause a drug's absorption to be reduced.[17] The net effect of these changes can be difficult to predict, and changes in drug absorption, caused by aging changes alone, may not be clinically significant. An elderly individual's absorption of a medication may be influenced by the way the medication is taken, what it is taken with, or by comorbid illnesses. For example, enteral feedings may interfere with the absorption of some medications (eg, phenytoin). Use of antacids, proton-pump inhibitors (ie, omeprazole), or H2 antagonists (ie, famotidine) increase gastric pH, thereby increasing the absorption of some drugs but decreasing the absorption of others.[3,18]

Distribution

The distribution of a medication refers to the location in the body that a drug penetrates and the time required for the medication to reach these locations. Older adults have an increase in body fat; thus, fat-soluble medications may have an increased volume of distribution, and they may also take longer to be eliminated from the body. Older adults also have decreased total body water; thus, medications that are water soluble (hydrophilic) may have a lower volume of distribution. Hypoalbuminemia (low blood protein stores) is not a normal condition of aging but is a common finding in the elderly. The levels of medications that are highly protein bound (eg, diazepam, phenytoin, and warfarin) can quickly become elevated or even toxic in patients with low protein stores. When caring for a patient with hypoalbuminemia, the nurse should assess for signs and symptoms of toxicity of any highly protein-bound medications that the patient is taking.

Metabolism

The most common site of drug metabolism is the liver. Given the normal aging changes of decreased hepatic blood flow and decreased hepatic size and mass, the older adult's hepatic metabolism of medications is reduced. This reduction may lead to elevated concentrations of medications in the body and, thus, ADEs. For example, in older adults, there is an approximately 60% reduction in the metabolism of NSAIDS and anticoagulant agents.[19] Given the potential for an increased concentration and duration of these medications, an elderly patient taking this medication combination has an elevated risk of gastrointestinal bleeding.

Elimination

Most medications are eliminated through the kidneys. Kidney function starts to decline in the fourth decade of life. Many older adults have some degree of renal compromise; thus, medications may take longer to be cleared from the body, and there is a higher risk of toxicity. A patient's estimated glomerular filtration rate should be taken into account when prescribing medications that are renally eliminated. Renally eliminated medication dosages and frequencies should be adjusted in the presence of kidney disease.

Pharmacodynamics and Aging

Pharmacodynamics is defined as what a mediation does to the body or how the body responds to the medication. The aging body's loss of cell function influences pharmacodynamics of medications, typically causing older adults to be more sensitive to medications. For example, elderly patients are very sensitive to medications with anticholinergic side effects (ie, antihistamines, urinary antimuscarinic agents, over-the-counter cold preparations) and may display concerning central nervous system adverse effects such as confusion and acute mental status changes when given these medications.

Iatrogenic Problems

Iatrogenic problems are side effects that are caused by a medication or treatment. Although iatrogenic side effects are not necessarily ADEs, they may contribute to them (see later discussion), and they could also contribute to an older adult's discomfort. Some classes of medications cause predictable iatrogenic problems. For example, opioid analgesics often cause constipation. The bedside nurse should be aware of common iatrogenic problems related to medications and monitor older patients for these. In addition to administering any ordered pharmaceuticals for these issues, nurses should maximize the use of nonpharmacologic interventions.

Consequences of Polypharmacy

Adverse drug event

An ADE is an injury that results from use of a medication. Risk factors for ADEs in older adults have been well documented (**Table 2**). ADEs are often categorized as drug-drug interactions or drug-disease interactions. Older adults are vulnerable to

Table 2
Risk factors of adverse drug events in the elderly

Patient Factors	Health Care System Factors
Age >85 y	Multiple prescribers
Frailty	Multiple pharmacies
Low body weight or body mass index	No regular reviews of patient's medication list
Six or more chronic health conditions	Poor communication among providers
Memory problems	Prescription of complex medical regimens
Estimated CrCl <50 mL/min	
9 + medications (prescribed and over the counter)	
12 + doses of medications/d	
Prior ADE	

Data from Administration on Aging. A profile of older Americans: 2015. 2015. Available at: https://aoa.acl.gov/Aging_Statistics/Profile/2015/docs/2015-Profile.pdf. Accessed December 20, 2016; and Mallet L, Spinewine A, Huang A. The challenge of managing drug interactions in elderly people. Lancet 2007;370(9582):185–91.

drug-drug interactions, as they often take multiple medications for their chronic health conditions. The risk of an ADE caused by drug-drug interactions increases with polypharmacy.[20,21] ADEs also occur when some medications are taken by patients with particular diseases. For example, patients with dementia have an increased sensitivity to medications with anticholinergic side effects and may exhibit acute mental status changes or delirium.

Approximately 4.3 million health care visits were attributed to ADEs in 2005.[22] Up to 35% of community-dwelling older adults have experienced an ADE that was discovered during an outpatient visit, and 40% of hospitalized older adults have experienced an ADE as well.[23] In 2013 to 2014, an estimated 34.5% of emergency department visits related to ADEs occurred among older adults, with anticoagulants, antibiotics, and diabetes agents being responsible for an estimated 46.9% of these visits.[24] Common drug classes associated with ADEs include anticoagulants, NSAIDs, cardiovascular medications, diuretics, antibiotics, anticonvulsants, benzodiazepines, and hypoglycemic medications.[23,25,26]

Older adults are at an increased risk of ADEs given the pharmacokinetic and pharmacodynamic changes that come with aging. Some ADEs are preventable, whereas others can be more difficult to predict. Common ADEs in older adults can be found in **Table 3**. Many ADEs are dose related, with higher dosages of medications carrying a higher risk.[27] Patients are the highest risk of having an ADE soon after starting a medication, but ADEs also may occur after a medication dosage increase is prescribed.

Costs
ADEs can cause unnecessary emergency department visits and hospitalizations, which contributes to increased health care costs for the patient and the health care system. Polypharmacy has also been associated with an increased risk of outpatient visits, hospitalizations, and emergency department visits.[24,28] Furthermore, polypharmacy may also contribute to rising out-of-pocket payment for medications.

PREVENTION OF POLYPHARMACY

Because of the risks and burden that polypharmacy and potentially inappropriate medications (PIMs) pose to patients and the health care system, it is incumbent on

Table 3 Common drug classes associated with adverse drug events	
Drug Class	**Common ADEs**
Anticoagulants	Bleeding/ulceration
Antipsychotics	Falls Parkinsonism Sedation
NSAIDs	Bleeding/ulceration Kidney impairment
Cardiovascular medications	Falls Decreased heart rate Hypotension Depression Hyperkalemia
Diuretics	Falls Hypotension Hypo/hyperkalemia SIADH/hyponatremia
Anticonvulsants	Sedation Falls SIADH/hyponatremia
Benzodiazepines	Falls Delirium Depression Sedation
Hypoglycemic medications	Falls Extreme hypoglycemia

Abbreviation: SIADH, syndrome of inappropriate antidiuretic hormone secretion.

interdisciplinary health care providers to use patient-centered approaches to optimize patient function and quality of life, reducing the use of PIMs when possible. Health care workers also have the opportunity to empower patients via knowledge and supportive interventions to use prescribed and over-the-counter agents appropriately.

Health Care Providers

Health care providers have the opportunity to assist in minimizing the use of PIMs. There are a variety of standardized, evidence-based tools available to guide health care providers in making pharmacologic decisions that meet the needs of older adults. Some tools such as the Beers Criteria, the screening tool of older people's prescriptions (STOPP), and screening tool to alert to right treatment (START) criteria condense medication-specific guidance.[29] Other frameworks, such as Scott's deprescribing framework, advise a patient-centered approach.[30] Medication-specific and patient-centered approaches may complement one another and can be used concurrently.

Beers Criteria

Initially published in 1991, the Beers Criteria was a list of medications that were potentially inappropriate for use in the elderly.[27] Today it is a rigorous clinical practice guideline published by a panel of experts who have conducted a comprehensive evidence review to identify medications that may confer additional risk to older adults.[30] The list additionally includes medications that may be inappropriate for older adults who have certain diseases or syndromes, such as avoidance of NSAID agents and thiazolidinediones in persons with heart failure.[29] A list of medications that may be used in older adults, but with which particular caution may be indicated, such as several anticoagulants, is also included.[30] A new addition in 2015 was tables of drug-drug interactions and medications with renal considerations that are pertinent to older adults.[30]

The authors of the current guidelines advise that the evidence-based lists provided are not intended to be used without clinician oversight.[27] Rather than using the Beers Criteria as a checklist, the authors advise incorporating the guidance into each patient's individualized plan of care, taking into account potential risks and benefits of each of their medications.[27]

Screening tool to alert to right treatment/screening tool of older people's prescriptions criteria

The STOPP/START criteria are similar to the Beers Criteria in that they include a list of medications that clinicians should consider avoiding or stopping on the STOPP list.[29] It also includes a START list of medications to consider applying in older adults based on evidence for improved outcomes.[29] Unlike the Beers Criteria, the STOPP/START criteria were drafted to be able to be used as a checklist.[29,30] This makes use of the STOPP/START criteria uniquely quick, and for this reason, it is often selected as a component of protocols for research or practice.

Deprescribing

In contrast to medication-centered approaches such as the Beers Criteria and START/STOPP criteria, a patient-centered deprescribing framework has been proposed as a novel method for considering an older adult's comprehensive health and medication list with specific attention to reducing PIMs.[31] This framework suggests that clinicians begin by ascertaining all of a patients' current medications—a simple-sounding task that can actually be challenging, particularly in the context of recent care transitions.[31] Clinicians should consider life expectancy and care goals when approaching a patient's medication list.[31] Each medication's benefits and harms should be weighed individually, incorporating evidence about similar older adults whenever possible.[31] In subsequent writings, Scott and colleagues[1] suggested a stepwise approach to deprescribing that provides clinicians with a structured process for considering relative risks and benefits. The term *deprescribing* is now used more broadly to connote not only Scott's framework but all efforts to reduce total number of medications and number of PIMs.

Implementation

There are several periods during care of older adults that may be opportunities for consideration of reduction of polypharmacy through use of either a medication-specific or patient-centered tool or both. Using evidence-based strategies to reduce PIMs should be considered during care transitions (eg, from hospital to home, from home to nursing facility), as care transitions are known to be a common juncture for medication errors. Hospitalization may be another appropriate time to reduce PIMs and to consider whether any of the patients' medications could have contributed to their hospital admission. Periods of relative stability when patients are following up with primary care providers represent another opportunity to intervene. Primary providers' long relationships with patients make them excellent candidates to engage in patient-centered methods that take into account the whole person and the person's care goals.

Significant variability exists in both rates of implementation and methods of deprescribing among health care providers. Some studies found that the incorporation of geriatric principles into health care education may increase rates of deprescribing.[32–34] Continuing education that includes content about deprescribing frameworks may also contribute to increased use of deprescribing principles.[35] Prompts embedded within an electronic health record may reduce the use of PIMs.[32]

Although there are several frameworks that may guide deprescribing efforts, selection of specific tools used is up to the individual provider.[35] This gives providers significant flexibility, but it may also contribute to confusion or lack of attention to deprescribing, as there is not a single standard of care. Some studies have found adoption of a single protocol on a unit or in a facility to be useful for reducing PIMs.[36,37]

Interestingly, although studies implementing deprescribing principles fairly consistently show a reduction in total number of medications and number of PIMs, there is a paucity of studies showing that these reductions in medications translate to reduced hospitalizations, rehospitalizations, or emergency department visits.[36,38,39] However, evidence about implementation of deprescribing frequently suggests that the most successful approaches may involve multiple disciplines working together for practice change.[32,36,40]

Patient communication

As clinicians apply frameworks to reduce PIMs, communication may be central to successful implementation. A study of older Italian adults found that 89% would prefer to take fewer medications.[41] However, patients and their loved ones are likely to lack an understanding of specific benefits and harms of each medication and will therefore rely on knowledgeable care providers to initiate communication about deprescribing.[42]

Conversations about medications should begin by listening to patients' concerns, preferences, and goals of care. Heath care workers can also listen for signs of unwanted side effects or adverse drug effects. After hearing patients' needs, providers may incorporate evidence-based knowledge about medications to make decisions. Communicating those decisions, along with pertinent rationales, may promote understanding of and adherence to suggested medication adjustments.

Reeve and colleagues[43] note that continuously re-informing patients about the relative risks and benefits of their medications as they age can be viewed as an ethical consideration. The omission of such conversations may be considered an ethical oversight and should compel clinicians to undertake deprescribing conversations with greater frequency.[43]

The role of the registered nurse

Registered nurses have many opportunities to facilitate deprescribing to reduce polypharmacy in older adults. Because nurses view patients holistically to provide individualized, cost-effective care, nurses may be particularly well equipped to intervene to reduce use of PIMs.

Nurses have the opportunity to promote the use of nonpharmacologic strategies to treat common symptoms such as sleeplessness, constipation, and behavioral symptoms of dementia. By using evidence-based nonpharmacologic strategies, nurses may be able to prevent the addition of medications such as sedatives or stool softeners. In addition to intervening with individual patients, nurses may also lead initiatives on their units or in their facilities to promote increased use of nonpharmacologic interventions across groups of patients.

In their role as direct care providers, nurses may have the opportunity to identify ADEs. By elevating concerns about potential ADEs, nurses may prompt conversations about deprescribing. Bringing knowledge of polypharmacy, its associated adverse outcomes, and specific frameworks for deprescribing (eg, Beers criteria, STOPP/ START criteria) may enhance the effectiveness of communication with prescribers.

Nurses are often, formally or informally, in the position of being intermediaries or co- ordinators between various care providers and in this role may have the opportunity to intervene on behalf of patients to ensure medication safety.[44] Nurses may have oppor- tunities to clarify medication lists, ensuring that intended medications are included and all other agents (eg, recently discontinued agents, agents intended only for short term use) are excluded. This may be a particularly complex and time-consuming task dur- ing care transitions.

Finally, nurses have the opportunity to lead initiatives aiming to educate interdisci- plinary team members and patients on improved medication management prac- tices.[45] Nurses can lead quality improvement projects to identify rates of polypharmacy in their care settings and to implement measures to improve rates of medication reconciliation and discontinuation of inappropriate medications.

Patients

Because older adults may take multiple medications and may have frequent medica- tion adjustments, patients may benefit from the use of interventions designed to pro- mote correct medication use. Because of normal changes of aging such as decline in visual acuity, accurate use of medications may be challenging for older adults. Nurses can encourage the use of in-home systems to promote accurate medication taking, and they can also facilitate in-person methods of reconciling and educating patients about their medications.

Medication management interventions

Numerous behavioral interventions to promote medication adherence exist, including reminders such as alarms or calendars, large-print labels, packaging/pillbox orga- nizers with medications presorted, and individual or group educational sessions.[46] A Cochrane Review to assess the relative efficacy of these strategies is ongoing.[46] Nurses may work with patients and pharmacists to select strategies that address each patient's unique needs.

Brown bag method

The brown bag method is a means of reviewing a patient's current medications that is often used by health care providers and pharmacists.[47] The aim of the brown bag medication review is to clarify a patient's current medication use and identify oppor- tunities to optimize their medication knowledge and use.[47]

A brown bag review begins by asking a patient to bring all of their current medica- tions, including over-the-counter and herbal agents, to their health care visit. The term brown bag references the idea that patients could bring all of their bottles in a brown bag or similar receptacle. The nurse or health care provider can then review medica- tions one at a time, reconciling each agent with the patient's medication list in the elec- tronic health record and querying patients' knowledge of correct administration and indication for each agent. The review serves as an opportunity to clarify a patient's medication list and to educate the patient about correct medication use.

SUMMARY

Polypharmacy is a growing problem in the United States and demands the attention of the registered nurse. Nurses in all health care settings have opportunities to reduce and prevent polypharmacy through implementation of evidence-based practices and delivery of person-centered care.

REFERENCES

1. Scott IA, Hilmer SN, Reeve E, et al. Reducing inappropriate polypharmacy: the process of deprescribing. JAMA Intern Med 2015;175(5):827–34.
2. Administration on Aging. A profile of older Americans: 2015. 2015. Available at: https://aoa.acl.gov/Aging_Statistics/Profile/2015/docs/2015-Profile.pdf. Accessed December 20, 2016.
3. Semla TP. Pharmacotherapy. In: Flaherty E, Resnick B, editors. Geriatric nursing review syllabus: a core curriculum in advanced practice geriatric nursing. 4th edition. New York: American Geriatrics Society; 2014. p. 81–9.
4. Gnjidic D, Hilmer SN, Blyth FM, et al. High-risk prescribing and incidence of frailty among older community-dwelling men. Clin Pharmacol Ther 2012;91(3):521–8.
5. Doshi JA, Shaffer T, Briesacher BA. National estimates of medication use in nursing homes: findings from the 1997 medicare current beneficiary survey and the 1996 medical expenditure survey. J Am Geriatr Soc 2005;53(3):438–43.
6. Dwyer LL, Han B, Woodwell DA, et al. Polypharmacy in nursing home residents in the United States: results of the 2004 national nursing home survey. Am J Geriatr Pharmacother 2010;8(1):63–72.
7. Saraf AA, Petersen AW, Simmons SF, et al. Medications associated with geriatric syndromes and their prevalence in older hospitalized adults discharged to skilled nursing facilities. J Hosp Med 2016;11(10):694–700.
8. Institute of Medicine. Preventing medication errors. 2006. Available at: http://www.nationalacademies.org/hmd/~/media/Files/Report%20Files/2006/Preventing-Medication-Errors-Quality-Chasm-Series/medicationerrorsnew.ashx. Accessed December 20, 2016.
9. Aitkens M, Valkova S. Avoidable costs in U.S. healthcare: the $200 billion opportunity from using medicines more responsibly. Parsippany (NJ): IMS Institute for Healthcare Informatics; 2013. Available at: http://www.imshealth.com/files/web/IMSH%20Institute/Reports/Avoidable_Costs_in%20_US_Healthcare/IHII_AvoidableCosts_2013.pdf. Accessed December 20, 2016.
10. Nishtala PS, Salahudeen MS. Temporal trends in polypharmacy and hyperpolypharmacy in older New Zealanders over a 9-year period: 2005-2013. Gerontology 2015;61(3):195–202.
11. Rochon PA, Gurwitz JH. Optimising drug treatment for elderly people: the prescribing cascade. BMJ 1997;315(7115):1096–9.
12. Tsiropoulos I, Andersen M, Hallas J. Adverse events with use of antiepileptic drugs: a prescription and event symmetry analysis. Pharmacoepidemiol Drug Saf 2009;18(6):483–91.
13. Caughey GE, Roughead EE, Pratt N, et al. Increased risk of hip fracture in the elderly associated with prochlorperazine: is a prescribing cascade contributing? Pharmacoepidemiol Drug Saf 2010;19(9):977–82.
14. Gill SS, Mamdani M, Naglie G, et al. A prescribing cascade involving cholinesterase inhibitors and anticholinergic drugs. Arch Intern Med 2005;165(7):808–13.
15. Kalisch LM, Caughey GE, Barratt JD, et al. Prevalence of preventable medication-related hospitalizations in Australia: an opportunity to reduce harm. Int J Qual Health Care 2012;24(3):239–49.
16. Kaufman G. Polypharmacy: the challenge for nurses. Nurs Stand 2016;30(39): 52–8.
17. Wooten JM. Pharmacotherapy considerations in elderly adults. South Med J 2012;105(8):437–45.

18. Kapadia A, Wynn D, Salzman B. Potential adverse effects of proton pump inhibitors in the elderly. Clin Geriatr 2010;18(7):24–31.
19. Wiffen P, Mitchell M, Snelling M, et al. Oxford handbook of clinical pharmacy. Oxford (England): University Press; 2007.
20. Field TS, Gurwitz JH, Avorn J, et al. Risk factors for adverse drug events among nursing home residents. Arch Intern Med 2001;161(13):1629–34.
21. Lu WH, Wen YW, Chen LK, et al. Effect of polypharmacy, potentially inappropriate medications and anticholinergic burden on clinical outcomes: a retrospective cohort study. Can Med Assoc J 2015;187(4):E130–7.
22. Bourgeois FT, Shannon MW, Valim C, et al. Adverse drug events I the outpatient setting: an 11-year national analysis. Pharmacoepidemiol Drug Saf 2010;19(9):901–10.
23. Hohl CM, Dankoff J, Colacone A, et al. Polypharmacy, adverse drug-related events, and potential adverse drug interactions in elderly patients presenting to an emergency department. Ann Emerg Med 2001;38(6):666–71.
24. Shehab N, Lovegrove MC, Gellar AI, et al. US emergency department visits for outpatient adverse drug events, 2013-2014. JAMA 2016;316(20):2115–25.
25. Marum ZA, Amuan ME, Hanlon JT, et al. Prevalence of unplanned hospitalizations caused by adverse drug reaction in older veterans. J Am Geriatr Soc 2012;60(1):34–41.
26. Gurwitz JH, Field TS, Harrold LR, et al. Incidence and preventability of adverse drug events among older persons in the ambulatory setting. JAMA 2003;289(9):1107–16.
27. Steinman MA, Beizer JL, DuBeau CE, et al. How to use the American Geriatrics Society 2015 Beers criteria – A guide for patients, clinicians, health systems, and payors. J Am Geriatr Soc 2015;63:e1–7.
28. Akazawa M, Imai H, Igarashi A, et al. Potentially inappropriate medication use in elderly Japanese patients. Am J Geriatr Pharmacother 2010;8(2):146–60.
29. O'Mahony D, O'Sullivan D, Byrne S, et al. STOPP/START criteria for potentially inappropriate prescribing in older people: version 2. Age Ageing 2015;44:213–8.
30. American Geriatrics Society 2015 Beers Criteria Update Expert Panel. American Geriatrics Society 2015 updated Beers criteria for potentially inappropriate medication use in older adults. J Am Geriatr Soc 2015;63:2227–46.
31. Scott IA, Gray LC, Martin JH, et al. Minimizing inappropriate medications in older populations: a 10-step conceptual framework. Am J Med 2012;125:529–37.
32. Lavan AH, Gallagher PF, O'Mahony D. Methods to reduce prescribing errors in elderly patients with multimorbidity. Clin Interv Aging 2016;11:857–66.
33. Monroe T, Carter M, Parish A. A case study using the Beers list criteria to compare prescribing by family practitioners and geriatric specialists in a rural nursing home. Geriatr Nurs 2011;32(5):350–6.
34. Corbi G, Gambassi G, Pagano G, et al. Impact of an innovative educational strategy on medication appropriate use and length of stay in elderly patients. Medicine 2015;94(24):1–7.
35. Skinner M. A literature review: polypharmacy protocol for primary care. Geriatr Nurs 2015;36(5):367–71.
36. Campins L, Serra-Prat M, Gozalo I, et al. Randomized controlled trial of an intervention to improve drug appropriateness in community-dwelling polymedicated elderly people. Fam Pract 2017;34(1):36–42.
37. Urfer M, Elzi L, Dell-Kuster S, et al. Intervention to improve appropriate prescribing and reduce polypharmacy in elderly patients admitted to an internal medicine unit. PLoS One 2016;11(11):e0166359.

38. Cooper JA, Cadogan CA, Patterson SM, et al. Interventions to improve the appropriate use of polypharmacy in older people: a cochrane systematic review. BMJ Open 2015;5(12):e009235.
39. Johansson T, Abuzahra ME, Keller S, et al. Impact of strategies to reduce polypharmacy on clinically relevant endpoints: a systematic review and meta-analysis. Br J Clin Pharmacol 2016;82(2):532–48.
40. Lenander C, Bondesson A, Midlov P, et al. Healthcare system intervention for safer use of medicines in elderly patients in primary care- a qualitative study of the participants' perceptions of self-assessment, peer review feedback and agreement for change. BMC Fam Pract 2015;117(16):1–9.
41. Galazzi A, Lusignani M, Chiarelli MT, et al. Attitudes towards polypharmacy and medication withdrawal among older inpatients in Italy. Int J Clin Pharm 2016;38: 454–61.
42. Palagyi A, Keay L, Harper J, et al. Barricades and brickwalls- a qualitative study exploring perceptions of medication use and deprescribing in long-term care. BMC Geriatr 2016;16(15):1–11.
43. Reeve E, Denig P, Hilmer SN, et al. The ethics of deprescribing in older adults. J Bioeth Inq 2016;13(4):581–90. Available at: http://link.springer.com/article/10.1007%2Fs11673-016-9736-y. Accessed December 20, 2016.
44. Johansson-Pajala RM, Blomgren KJ, Bastholm-Rahmer P, et al. Nurses in municipal care of the elderly act as pharmacovigilant intermediaries: a qualitative study of medication management. Scand J Prim Health Care 2016;34(1):37–45.
45. Vejar MV, Makic MBF, Kotthoff-Burrell E. Medication management for elderly patients in an academic primary care setting: a quality improvement project. J Am Assoc Nurse Pract 2015;27:72–8.
46. Cross AJ, Elliott RA, George J. Interventions for improving medication-taking ability and adherence in older adults prescribed multiple medications. Cochrane Database Syst Rev 2016. http://dx.doi.org/10.1002/14651858.CD012419. Available at: http://onlinelibrary.wiley.com/doi/10.1002/14651858.CD012419/full. Accessed on December 27, 2016.
47. Nathan A, Goodyer L, Lovejoy A, et al. 'Brown bag' medication reviews as a means of optimizing patients' use of medication and of identifying potential clinical problems. Fam Pract 1999;16(3):278–82.

Impaired Mobility and Functional Decline in Older Adults

Evidence to Facilitate a Practice Change

 CrossMark

Deanna Gray-Miceli, PhD, GNP-BC, FAAN, FAANP, FGSA, FNAP[a,b],*

KEYWORDS

- Impaired mobility • Physician function • Older adults • Nagi disablement framework
- Lived experience • Geriatric syndromes

KEY POINTS

- Individualizing care to improve function and mobility is an essential component in the provision of quality health care to older adults.
- The overall health promotion effects of early intervention around a basic necessity, mobility, are clear.
- Untoward health outcomes from reduced mobility and functional decline are also well established.
- Professional nurses will need to advocate for older adults on their units in the hospital and in other settings, by critically analyzing policies and procedures, ensuring that mobility is properly assessed, and mobility impairment is addressed by all members of the health care team.

INTRODUCTION

On any day of the year, and instigated by many factors, impaired mobility and functional decline occur, all too commonly, among thousands of adults over the age of 65 in our nation.[1] Functional limitations, such as inability to ambulate and impaired mobility, are precursors to disability of notable clinical significance and importance to older adults. Not only are mobility limitations common in older adults and due to multiple determinants such as the effects of chronic diseases, but also mobility

The author reports no funding for this work, and no conflicts of interest.
^a Rutgers University, School of Nursing, 180 University Avenue, 258 Ackerson Hall, Newark, NJ 07102, USA; ^b Institute for Health, Health Care Policy and Aging Research, 112 Paterson Street, New Brunswick, NJ 08901, USA
* Corresponding author. Rutgers University, School of Nursing, 180 University Avenue, 258 Ackerson Hall, Newark, NJ 07102.
E-mail addresses: dmiceli@sn.rutgers.edu; deannanp@aol.com

limitation affects the physical, psychological, and social aspects of the their daily life.[2] Acute medical illness is also cited for their hospitalization-associated disability outcomes among older adults.[3] Although disability among older adults is not limited to the home, hospital, or institutional long-term care environment, evidence shows functional limitations can be recognized and prevented from progression.

Of all the likely health care providers, it is the registered professional nurse who is most likely to encounter a patient experiencing a functional decline and who is prepared with the appropriate education, knowledge, and clinical skill competency to do something about it. Moreover, according to the Institute of Medicine's *Future of Nursing* Report, it is the licensed professional nurse, for which there are 3.7 million, who are likely to "dominate in a reformed healthcare system as it inevitably moves toward an emphasis on prevention and management, rather than acute (hospital) care."[4]

The following exemplar, drawn from the lived experience of an 88-year-old retired nurse practitioner, and participant in doctoral dissertation research, was living quite content and comfortable with her husband of 50 years, reporting "good health and function," until a series of falls occurred. Periods of confinement and reduced mobility, teetering on the verge of immobility and isolation, were the aftermath of a fall for Molly.[5]

Molly's Lived Experience of a Serious Fall and the Role of the Nurse

"I thought, why this did happen, why did you have to spoil the trip? I say there I go again, then I slow down for a while (meaning I stay indoors, don't get up out of the chair, don't go outdoors). I see it as one more fall... oh no, now what's going to happen to me? I'm going to be more disabled sooner than I care to be. Falling, and not getting up again, means I have to make great adjustments (to my routine in daily living)... Slow Down! I can't go outside to the garden, which I love; my partner wants me to move faster than I can."[5]

Further inquiry revealed: "the nurses watch out for you here... she called and was worried it was several days and no Molly. She came to visit and made me get up out of that chair... go to therapy... notify the medical doctor... and go to the wellness center for activity. I've made progress, walking outdoors more and meeting friends for dinner at the dining room."

Dialogue between the professional nurse at the life care community and Molly illustrates the importance of advocacy and early intervention by the professional registered nurse as she recognized Molly's pattern change in mobility and function. The nurse then championed Molly toward improved mobility and function. Outcomes such as these are achievable by all professional nurses who care for an older adult clientele. It is important to recognize however, "the interaction between mobility, independence and well-being are contextual in older person's lives, and will differ between places, individuals and across phases in each individual's unique lifecourse."[6] Hence, a thorough understanding and examination by the professional nurse at the point of care of all intraindividual and extraindividual factors, which interact as determinants of mobility, are critical to assess.

The purpose of this article is to assist professional nurses in any practice environment to identify, prevent, and manage clinical characteristics and phenomena associated with impaired mobility, to properly assess, document, and communicate issues effecting mobility, to identify evidenced-based nursing care intervention strategies to help mitigate the progression of reduced mobility to immobility, and to gain insight from discovery of the older adult's perception of their reduced mobility based on lived experience so as to embrace their unique perspectives, wishes, and values in a patient-centered context of a caring, practice environment.

BACKGROUND AND SIGNIFICANCE

Reduced physical mobility and immobility have long been cited to belong to one of the shared risk factors comprising a "geriatric syndrome."[7] The 5 classic geriatric syndromes recognized in clinical care of the older adult, across all practice settings, include pressure ulcers, urinary incontinence, falls, functional decline, and delirium. Geriatric syndromes are unique in occurrence to the older adult population, and when recognized early and treated accordingly, their impact to the person and to health care expenditures can be lessened. The shared risk factors of impaired mobility and impaired function, which cocontribute to the development of the classic 5 types of geriatric syndromes, are significant predictors of longer hospital lengths of stay and repeat hospitalizations (impaired mobility:odds ratio = 1.94, $P<.001$, and impaired function:odds ratio = 1.68, $P<.01$, respectively).[8] Because geriatric syndromes are recognized as largely preventable,[7] the value of early recognition and treatment of impaired mobility and functional limitations by health care providers translate, at the individual level, to opportunities for older adults patients to achieve or improve wellness, functional independence, and overall quality of life.

Preventing physical impairments from becoming a functional limitation in daily living and/or a disability is a fundamental goal in the provision of quality care to all older adults supported by national health care initiatives.[9] Recognizing and planning care appropriately for older adults with impaired mobility and functional decline is critically important to alter the disablement process where an eventual outcome includes frailty.

Frailty not only increases risk to fall but also is an independent predictor of disability, hospitalization, iatrogenic complications, and mortality among older adults.[10–13] Clinical investigations of the frailty phenotype show unique characteristics, many of which are evident on physical assessment; these include loss of muscle mass, muscle weakness, poor endurance (or energy), slow gait speed, and low physical activity levels.[11] The conceptual definition of "frailty" involves the interaction of loss of muscle mass and functional independence in the face of chronic multiple diseases.[11]

In most all health care settings, but especially in the long-term care setting, it is the older adult patient, over the age of 85, with the greatest functional limitations and highest degree of disease burden, who is at greatest risk for impaired mobility.[14,15] In this practice environment, older adults are a vulnerable population with unique health needs. As such, health care must be provided by a competent and compassionate nursing workforce poised to adequately address the unique needs of this population. The extent to which impaired mobility and function can be lessened will occur by "aggressively promoting public health interventions aimed at specifically closing the gaps in quality of care delivered to each patient through patient-centered care."[16]

Another high-risk practice environment where older adults experience impaired mobility and functional decline of new onset is the acute care hospital. Evidence shows the onset of functional decline can occur in a matter of days.[17] As such, reducing functional decline in older adults has received much attention by researchers, clinical scholars, and national nursing policy experts in acute and critical care.[18] Fundamental aspects to enhance function among hospitalized older adults include creating a culture of care framework with goals to (1) promote recovery; (2) optimize reserve; (3) maintain safety; (4) support independence; (5) uphold dignity; (6) maintain vigilance; (7) cultivate responsiveness; and (8) improve access.[18]

RECOGNITION OF IMPAIRED MOBILITY AND FUNCTIONAL DECLINE WITHIN A CONCEPTUAL FRAMEWORK

Assessment and care planning for the older adult to achieve or maintain peak quality of life is a universal goal of care providers of older adults, in every encounter, and in any practice setting. Quality-of-life determinations by older adults are often situationally influenced, from both intraindividual and extraindividual factors, including such events as the development of a functional impairment, which can ultimately limit the person's function, resulting in a disability. It has long been clinically recognized within the Nagi Disablement Framework, organ or body system level factors, such as pathologic diseases resulting in physical impairments, such as reduced muscular strength, can lead to a functional limitation characterized by the older adult's inability to perform the activity, such as walking or maintenance of mobility (**Fig. 1**).[19]

Functional limitations have implications for the older adult because they continue to perform customary roles within their families and society. Inability to fulfill family, spousal, and community roles, or even personal goals set by the individual, constitutes at the social level a disability of handicap.[19] According to the Nagi framework, it is the functional limitation, such as inability to shop, drive, or walk that directly impacts one's quality-of-life perceptions and rating as well as the inability to fulfill previously valued roles in society.[19]

Nursing assessment of the older adult's baseline level of physical function, related to mobility, provides a benchmark for restoration goal setting with the older adult. Thus, at the point of care, nurses must not only learn how to perform a functional assessment but also critically analyze all relevant intraindividual and extraindividual factors influencing mobility, such as past and current health status, symptoms experienced, and environment as they impact on the older adult's physical mobility, activity, and function (**Box 1**). As espoused in Melnyk and Fineout-Overholt's framework[20] for the context of caring using evidenced-based practices, applying this knowledge to the patient's wishes will help direct the selection of the best evidence-based practice intervention to use to restore physical mobility and function leading to quality patient outcomes.

Another theoretic framework for mobility, applicable to care of older adults, is the conical model of 7 life-space locations.[21] Mobility can be conceptualized to occur for older adults along 7 life-space locations, which include room, home, outdoors, neighborhood, service community, surrounding area, and world. The importance of recognizing mobility within these life-space locations is it provides for a conceptualization beyond the immediate location and health encounter between the nurse and the patient, which is often space constricted and confined to a single "patient" room.

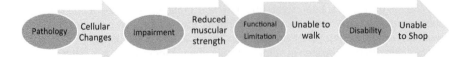

Fig. 1. Progression of disease to disability in the Nagi Disablement Framework for older adults. Application of symptoms from lived experience of a serious fall. (*Adapted from* Gray Miceli D, Ratcliffe SJ. Post-fall emotional responses, functional limitations and action plans to manage falls among independent residing older adults with recurrent falls. Gerontologist 2015;55(Suppl 2):644; and the Nagi Disablement Framework. Verbrugge LM, Jette AM. The disablement process. Soc Sci Med 1994;38(1):1–4.)

Box 1
Demographic, situational, and clinical determinants influencing mobility in older adults

Demographic factors:
  Over the age of 85

Intraindividual factors:
  History of recent lower extremity fracture
  History of recent falls, incontinence, pressure ulcer
  History of a serious fall, and emotional responses[a]
  Diagnosis of a geriatric syndrome
  History of chronic illnesses:
    Cognitive impairment
    Dementia
    Depression
    Diabetes
    Stroke
  Presence of gait or balance impairment
  Presence of visual impairment
  Presence of acute or chronic pain
  Presence of acute/chronic diseases with distressful symptoms; dizziness with standing from orthostatic hypotension; lightheadedness with head turning, vertigo[b]
  Presence of lower extremity pain/weakness
  Presence of foot pain from heel spur, bunion, callus, or other abnormality

Extraindividual factors[c]:
  Access to assistive devices or human help
  Access to and use of appropriate foot wear[d]
  Environmental safety:
    Neighborhood changes and crime[e]
    Condition of steps, sidewalk[e]
    Outdoor weather[e]

Situational factors:
  Recent sentinel event
  Recent acute care hospitalization
  Recent acute life-threatening illness: sepsis, traumatic brain injury, stroke
  Fear of falling
  Resident satisfaction with staff[f]
  Staff encouragement for physical activity[f]

Other factors:
  Frailty
  Polypharmacy/inappropriate medication use
  Adverse drug reaction causing fatigue, inertia, leg weakness, or other bothersome symptoms

[a] Gray-Miceli D, Ratcliffe SJ. Post-fall emotional responses, functional limitations and action plans to manage falls among independent residing older adults with recurrent falls. Gerontologist 2015;55(Suppl 2):644.
[b] Gray-Miceli D, Johnson, JC, Strumpf, NE. A stepwise approach to comprehensive post-fall assessment. Ann Long Term Care 2005;13(12):16–24.
[c] Gray-Miceli D. Step 3: detecting environmental hazards and modifying the environment for patient and healthcare worker safety. In: Five easy steps to prevent falls: the comprehensive guide for nurses to keeping patients of all ages safe. Silver Spring (MD): American Nurses Association; 2014. p. 90-102. Available at: http://www.nursesbooks.org/Homepage/Hot-off-the-Press/5-Easy-Steps-To-Prevent-Falls.aspx.
[d] Gray-Miceli D. Part I: falls in the environment: faulty footwear or footing?: interdisciplinary case-based perspectives. Ann Long Term Care 2010;18(4):32–6.
[e] Marquez DX, Aguinage S, Campa J, et al. A qualitative exploration of factors associated with walking and physical activity in community-dwelling older Latino adults. J Appl Gerontol 2016;35(6) 664–77.
[f] Holmes SD, Galik E, Resnick B. Factors that influence physical activity among residents in assisted living. J Gerontol Soc Work 2017;60(2):120–37.

According to this mobility theoretic framework, the key influencers of mobility at each level are broad and inclusive to include the multiple influences of cognitive, psychosocial, physical environmental, financial, as well as gender, culture, and biographic information.

Using both of these theoretic models simultaneously can help the nurse to envision the inherent progression of a functional impairment to disability within the older adult's life-space location. Functional limitations extend beyond "where one sleeps" to include the older adult's broader world of existence. When caring for older adults, nurses must consider the influence of the many intraindividual and extraindividual factors or determiners of mobility (see **Box 1**). Discovery of the impact of these factors is a necessary requirement in order to plan nursing care appropriately.

Among all of the factors illustrated in **Box 1**, least understood and researched are the emotional responses, aftermaths, and relationships to quality of life of each of these intraindividual, extraindividual, situational, and other factors. As way of example, exemplary care of older adults does not simply observe or attempt to reduce risk factors and determiners for these adverse events increasing risk for reduced mobility. Instead, gerontologic nurses seek to respond to the older adult's unique response to impaired mobility and functional decline through understanding the personal impact of these conditions in their lives. Active listening to older adults' stories and lived experience is one way to gain insight into the meaning this phenomena has in their life world. Moreover, although there is an exhaustive body of knowledge in the research literature in care of older adults related to both risks and outcomes of impaired physical mobility and functional decline, there is a paucity of evidence in the geriatric research literature detailing the personal accounts voiced by older adults themselves from lived experiences of reduced mobility.

RECOGNITION OF IMPAIRED MOBILITY AND FUNCTIONAL DECLINE FROM OLDER ADULTS' LIVED EXPERIENCES

In prior qualitative research, older adults voiced concern about the situational context they experienced following a fall perceived to be "serious."[5] These falls were perceived serious, not because of physical injury per se, but because they were life altering, resulting in confinement, and reduced mobility, with strong and sustained emotional responses.[5] Their quality of life was impacted as lives changed because of the new onset of functional limitations and disability (**Fig. 2**).[5] All of the independent and high-functioning community-dwelling participants (n = 19), with an average age of 83.3 years, experienced a *changed life* because of altered personal selves, altered functional selves, and altered social selves.[22] Their emotional responses, such as anger and frustration, feeling hopeless and helpless following their most serious fall, led to self-confinement indoors, reduced mobility, refusal to go outdoors to socialize (due to smashed noses and bruised faces), thus altering their social roles and social selves.[22]

Nursing assessment of the older adult for the presence or absence of impairments resulting in reduced mobility or functional limitation begins with exploration of the older adult's account of their lived experiences and self-perceptions of their current state of health, wellness, and overall function. At the start of the interview and assessment process on day 1 of the health care encounter, nurses begin by gathering important information from the health history of prior medical illness and symptoms related to these illnesses, medications used in the management of these conditions, and the resulting impact of the condition or disease resulting in impairment and/or functional limitation, if any (see **Box 1**).

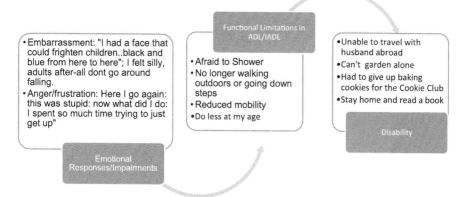

Fig. 2. Sample of older adults lived experience of a serious fall applied to the Nagi Disablement Framework. IADL, instrumental activities of daily living. (*Adapted from* Gray-Miceli D, Ratcliffe SJ. Post-fall emotional responses, functional limitations and action plans to manage falls among independent residing older adults with recurrent falls. Gerontologist 2015;55(Suppl 2):644.)

ASSESSMENT OF PHYSICAL FUNCTION: ACTIVITIES OF DAILY LIVING

Functional status is determined by the nurse in response to the older adult's ability to execute/perform basic activities of daily living (ADL) related to dressing, bathing, ambulation, eating, and toileting.[23] The classic measurement tools used to elicit the older adult's ability to perform basic ADLs is through self-report or from a proxy such as the family caregiver. Equally important, however, is the validation by the nurse of the patient's ADL function through observation of their ability to perform the task because this provides for true measures when subjective bias is minimized. Therefore, during periods of activity on the unit, or in the older adult's home, observation of performance in bathing, dressing, eating, and ambulation is the gold standard versus self-report. It is also during observation that the nurse can observe for any musculoskeletal, neurologic, vision, or balance impairments. Evidence suggests current Medicare beneficiaries over the age of 85 need more help with basic ADLs than those between the ages of 65 and 84 years (**Table 1**).[24] Of those individuals aged 85 and older who reported difficulty in the same year, 27.7% (25.2–30.1; n = 671,833) of individuals had difficulty getting the help they needed.[24]

ASSESSMENT OF AMBULATION AND MOBILITY

Ambulation is an important component to performing basic ADLs and important aspect of mobility. As illustrated in the conical 7 life-space conceptual framework, mobility is a broad concept that extends beyond the current situation where the nurse encounters the older adult, for instance, in the emergency department, hospital unit, or assisted living community.

Impaired mobility in its broadest sense means the older adult requires assistance of human or mechanical help to maintain upright mobility, so as to ambulate or walk, and in its strictest sense means the older adult is limited and/or confined in their ability to be freely mobile. Impaired mobility is a situation that results from the interaction of

Table 1
Percent of Medicare beneficiaries reporting difficulties with common activities and those getting help, by age group: 2012

	Beneficiaries Aged 65-84 Percent (95% confidence interval, CI)	Beneficiaries Aged 85 and Older Percent (95% CI)	Beneficiaries Aged 85 and Older Percent (95% CI) with Difficulty Getting Help	Frequency
Activities of Daily Living (ADL)				
Walking	24.5 (23.4–25.5)	50.5 (48.4–52.6)	27.7 (25.2–30.1)	671,833
Getting in/out of bed/chair	11.8 (11.1–12.6)	25.0 (23.1–26.9)	38.1 (34.0–42.1)	458,840
Bathing	8.6 (8.0–9.2)	25.8 (23.7–27.8)	68.4 (64.2–72.6)	848,363
Dressing	6.5 (6.0–7.1)	17.0 (15.3–18.8)	74.4 (69.4–79.5)	609,333
Toileting	4.4 (4.0–4.9)	12.8 (11.5–14.1)	46.5 (40.3–52.7)	286,335
Eating	2.9 (2.5–3.3)	6.9 (5.8–8.1)	46.7 (38.1–55.3)	155,531

From Centers for Medicare and Medicaid Services Releases: 2012 MCBS Access to Care Research Files: Are Medicare Beneficiaries Getting the Help They Need with Home-Based Care? Medicare Current Beneficiaries Survey. Data Brief #002, July 2014.

multiple factors at the person level of the unit level and so may be modifiable (see **Box 1**). It should be noted that many acute illnesses can be heralded by acute changes in function and mobility, and in many circumstances, because of their nature, are treatable, and thus, the unintended consequences of impaired or reduced mobility and functional decline can be modifiable. Unit-level factors include the availability and willingness of staff to access mobility aid or to help the older adult ambulate on a regular basis. Goals include the following: to forestall functional decline by addressing modifiable risk factors (see **Box 1**) and to promote early and continued upright mobility or ambulation. The consequences of impaired mobility need to be recognized and managed early so as to prevent long-term complications (**Box 2**) and to avoid iatrogenesis.[25]

Box 2
Consequences of untreated impaired mobility in older adults

Physical response to current limitation

- Skin breakdown and pressure ulcers
- Loss of calcium from bones, osteopenia/osteoporosis
- Joint contractures and joint pain
- Reduced and/or loss of muscle mass
- Reduced circulation
- Risk for infection (respiratory and genitourinary)
- Risk for reduced oral intake/dehydration
- Constipation/fecal impaction

Functional response to current limitation[a]

- Self-care neglect due to inability to carry out activities of daily living
- Dependency on others to assist in activities of daily living
- Functional limitation in activities of daily living
- Functional limitations in instrumental activities of daily living

Emotional response to current limitation[a]

- Angry/frustrated
- Feeling helpless
- Feeling hopeless
- Fear of becoming "disabled"
- Feeling ashamed; embarrassment

Social response to current limitation[a]

- Bed, chair, institutional, or home confinement
- Familial or societal role changes: inability to carry out usual role
- Becoming dependent on others

[a] *Data from* Gray-Miceli D, Ratcliffe SJ. Post-fall emotional responses, functional limitations and action plans to manage falls among independent residing older adults with recurrent falls. Gerontologist 2015;55(Suppl 2):644; and Gray-Miceli D. Changed life: a phenomenological study of the meaning of serious falls to older adults, Widener University; 2001 (UMI Microform No. 3005877).

Health History

The ability to maintain upright mobility is contingent upon intact interfunctioning of the central and peripheral nervous systems, the sensory and visual systems, and the musculoskeletal system. Assessment of cognitive, neurologic, and sensory factors affecting mobility begins with a detailed review of systems for factors involved in the nursing assessment of the musculoskeletal system related to ambulation and mobility in older adults (**Box 3**).

Older adults with intact central, peripheral nervous systems, sensory and musculo-skeletal systems may have difficulty with mobility, because of chronic illnesses and/or medications taken to manage these diseases. For this reason, it is important in the assessment of mobility to review questions during the health encounter that may indicate the older adult has a potential for impairment in mobility. For each positive response elicited, the professional nurse needs to further determine the onset, duration, timing, severity, aggravating and alleviating factors, and how these symptoms impact on not only overall mobility but also overall function. It is vital to not only elicit this information but also frame the plan of care and communication with the physician or nurse practitioner accordingly. Begin the series of questions about mobility concentrating on the musculoskeletal system (see **Box 3**).

Physical Assessment

Following a detailed review of systems, the nurse progresses to physical assessment of the musculoskeletal and neurologic systems (**Box 4**).

Correlating positive responses from the health history with the physical assessment is paramount to detect impaired mobility. The physical examination of the older adult begins with the older adult lying supine in bed. The nurse begins the physical assessment by inspection, followed by palpation and range of motion of the muscles and joints, noting abnormalities (see **Box 4**).

Clinical Decision Making About Safety to Ambulate

Once the health history and physical examination of the musculoskeletal, neurologic, sensory system, and mobility have been gathered, the nurse should make an informed determination: *Is it prudent and safe to administer aids to quantitatively rate the older person's physical mobility performance, which entail having the patient stand and/or ambulate independently?* For safety reasons, it may be advisable to have another nurse standing close by, so as to avoid any potential accidental falls when the older adult is asked to stand upright. This determination is made by the primary professional nurse, on an individual case-by-case basis, according to the person's ability to understand what is being asked and to be capable of performing the activity. The older adult patient may be too weak or fatigued or exhibit reduced muscle weakness in the lower extremities to stand, even with help. It is also vital to ascertain the patient preferences and wishes, taking into consideration their goals and individual needs.

It is also critical to note that it is not safe for the nurse to assess the older patient's gait or standing balance if they are experiencing states of extreme muscle weakness, hemiparesis, or cognitive impairment such as delirium or sedation.

SELECTED MEASUREMENT SCALES TO DETERMINE MOBILITY AND BALANCE

There are several measures to quantitate mobility among older adults. Some of the measures also incorporate both static and dynamic balance determination. Therefore, it may be indicated for the nurse to first assess if a balance impairment exists. In addition to observation of balance impairments, the patient may indicate they have

Box 3
Sample review of systems questions involved in the nursing assessment of ambulation and mobility safety in older adults

General

Do you experience any periods of fatigue or weakness that limit your walking?

Have you noticed any changes in your mobility over the past month?

If your mobility has changed, when did you notice this change? Do you think it was related to a recent fall? Injury? Medication? Or following hospital discharge?

After you walk a few steps, do you feel the need to sit down and rest?

Vision

Do you have any blurry or double vision? How is your vision? Do you use corrective lenses? Do you think your vision is adequate for seeing your environment to ambulate safely?

Hips/knees/spine/feet

Do you experience joint discomfort or pain in your hips, knees, spine, or feet with standing or walking? Do you experience any lower leg weakness? In one leg or both legs? When did you notice this change? Was it related to a recent fall? Medication? Or event such as being discharged from the hospital?

Do you experience any lower leg weakness when you weight bear or stand up?

Do you take pain medications for the pain? If so, has it helped?

Balance

How is your balance while sitting? While standing? Or getting up? While walking?

Do you experience any difficulty or use any aids to help with balance?

Shoe-wear

Do you normally walk with your shoes on or do you walk with slippers or bare feet?

Are you able to walk, unassisted, wearing your shoes?

Describe your current shoe-wear: ideally shoes should be rubber soled, leather, laced up or with Velcro fasteners that fit snug and are not loose; they should have ankle support and they should have a wedged heel.

Use of human or mechanical assistive device

Are you able to stand up, unassisted, from a seated position or do you require assistance; for instance, do you use arm rails? Or do you need the help of a person?

Once you are standing, are you able to take a few steps and walk without assistance?

Do you currently need the help of a person, such as arm- in-arm assistance, to keep you upright while you are walking?

Do you currently need the help of a device such as a straight cane or walking aid to maintain your upright balance while walking?

Do you currently hold on to furniture or the wall while you are walking?

Physical activity

What type of physical activity or exercise do you enjoy? How often do you perform this activity? Do you perform yoga? Tai chi? Or sports such as swimming? Walking? Running? Tennis?

Data from Gray-Miceli D. Step 1: eliciting a fall focused health history. In: Five easy steps to prevent falls: the comprehensive guide for nurses to keeping patients of all ages safe. Silver Spring (MD): American Nurses Association; 2014. p. 36–41. Available at: http://www.nursesbooks.org/Homepage/Hot-off-the-Press/5-Easy-Steps-To-Prevent-Falls.aspx.

Box 4
Physical assessment of the musculoskeletal and neurologic system

Patient is lying supine in bed

Inspect: Are the muscles of the lower legs and thighs similar in size symmetrically?
  Is there evidence of atrophy or muscle wasting?
  Is there joint swelling or fluid evident of the knee?
  Do the joints feel hot or warm to touch?
  Is there any redness of the joints or muscles?
  Are there bruises around the hip or knee joints or pelvis?

Inquire: Is the older adult able to perform a straight leg-raising test, one leg at a time?
  Are they able to do this? Or is there difficulty or an impairment in one leg?

Assess muscular strength by placing your hands on the soles of the patient's feet; ask them to push:
  Is there equal strength in both feet when pushed against your hand?
  Assess dorsi and plantar flexion and extension and note findings.

Assess passive range of motion: Bend the patients knee (one at a time) while cupping the examiner's hand over the knee to perform passive range of motion
  Do you note any crepitus or limitation of the knee with this maneuver?
  Is there restricted range of motion or is the range of motion normal?

Inspect the ankles and toes noting any redness, inflammation, corns, calluses, or bunions

Assess position sense of the great toe bilaterally, note symmetry

Assess vibratory sense over bony prominences bilaterally, note symmetry

Assess touch sensation of the lower legs with the patient's eyes closed

Assess lower extremity deep tendon reflexes

Assess temperature and pin prick sensation to very cold objects and sharp objects

Patient is sitting on the bed or is sitting in a straight-back chair

Assess: Is the patient able to raise their leg straight up with their knee bent against your hand; as you press down, is there evidence of muscle weakness in either leg?

---

experienced a loss of balance or balance impairment. Falls can be an indication of balance impairment, even if the patient does not indicate they experience balance difficulties. Most often in the health care setting, the older adult can be referred for an occupational and/or physical therapy evaluation to formally quantitate both gait and balance impairments. Before beginning the actual performance of these balance tests with an occupational or physical therapist, as needed, it is preferred that the nurse gauges the older person's perception of their own confidence in ADLs. For this reason, the Falls Efficacy Scale (FES)[26] should be used following the health history appraisal.

The Falls Efficacy Scale

The FES is a measure of an older adult's self-rated confidence in their ability to perform routine activities such as those within the domain of ADL. The scale is administered by the nurse at the bedside and includes 10 questions, each rated along a scale of 1 to 10. One indicates, "I am very confident to do this activity," whereas a score of 10 indicates, "I am not confident at all." This test takes less than 5 minutes to administer and can provide a quick gauge of the person's perception of their abilities. The authors indicate a score greater than 70 indicates the person has a fear of falling (**Table 2**).[26]

Table 2 Falls efficacy scale	
Name:	Date:
On a scale from 1 to 10, with 1 being very confident and 10 being not confident at all, how confident are you that you do the following activities without falling?	
Activity:	Score: 1 = very confident 10 = not confident at all
Take a bath or shower	
Reach into cabinets or closets	
Walk around the house	
Prepare meals not requiring carrying heavy or hot objects	
Get in and out of bed	
Answer the door or telephone	
Get in and out of a chair	
Get dressed and undressed	
Personal grooming (ie, washing your face)	
Get on and off of the toilet	
Total score	

A total score of greater than 70 indicates that the person has a fear of falling.
   Data from "Timed Up and Go (TUG)". Minnesota Falls Prevention. Available at: http://www.mnfallsprevention.org/professional/riskresearch.html. Accessed June 9, 2017; and Tinetti ME, Richman D, Powell L. Falls efficacy as a measure of fear of falling. J Gerontol 1990;45(6):P239.

The 30-second Chair Stand Test

The 30-second chair stand test balance motion is actually an industry standard assessment used by clinicians in their assessment of an older adult's balance, as recommended by the Centers for Disease Control and Prevention in their STEADI (Stopping Elderly Accidents, Deaths and Injuries) Toolkit for practitioners. During the sit-to-stand maneuver, subjects are timed using a stopwatch. Subjects are given 30 seconds to perform this maneuver, and they may use the armrest on the chair to help themselves up if needed. The sit to stand (STS) test is illustrated in **Fig. 3**.[27]

Berg Balance Scale

The Berg Balance Scale-14 has been developed to measure balance among older people with impairment in balance function, by assessing the performance of functional tasks. It consists of a 5-point dichotomous scale ranging from 0 to 4, where "0" indicates the lowest level of function and "4" indicates higher functioning. Its major barrier is that it is only measuring balance at one specific point in time, and thus, for activities such as walking a straight line, potential risks to subjects will not be identified.[28]

Timed Up and Go Test

The Timed Up and Go test is used to measure both static and dynamic (walking) balance. It measures the time it takes for the subject to rise from the chair, walk 3 m, turn around, and walk back to the chair and sit down. The longer it takes to perform this test of mobility, the greater the likelihood the person needs assistance with mobility and the more likely they are to be at risk for falls. Scores of 10 seconds or less indicate

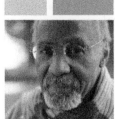

Patient: _____   Date: _____   Time: _____   AM/PM

The 30-S Chair Stand Test

Purpose: To test leg strength and endurance

Equipment:

- A chair with a straight back without arm rests (seat 17" high)
- A stopwatch

Instructions to the patient:

1. Sit in the middle of the chair.
2. Place your hands on the opposite shoulder crossed at the wrists.
3. Keep your feet flat on the floor.
4. Keep your back straight and keep your arms against your chest.
5. On **"Go,"** rise to a full standing position and then sit back down again.
6. Repeat this for 30 s.

On **"Go,"** begin timing.

If the patient must use his/her arms to stand, stop the test. Record "0" for the number and score.

Count the number of times the patient comes to a full standing position in 30 s.

If the patient is over halfway to a standing position when 30 s have elapsed, count it as a stand.

Record the number of times the patient stands in 30 s.

Number: _____   Score_____   See next page.

A below average score indicates a high risk for falls.

Notes:

For relevant articles, go to: **www.cdc.gov/injury/STEADI**

Chair Stand—Below Average Scores

Age	Men	Women
60–64	<14	<12
65–69	<12	<11
70–74	<12	<10
75–79	<11	<10
80–84	<10	<9
85–89	<8	<8
90–94	<7	<4

Fig. 3. The 30-second chair stand test. (*From* CDC. STEADI- Older Adult Falk Prevention. Available at: https://www.cdc.gov/steadi/pdf/30_second_chair_stand_test-a.pdf.)

normal mobility, whereas scores between 11 and 20 are within normal limits for frail elders and those disabled, and scores greater than 20 seconds indicate the older adult needs further ambulation assistance and intervention. Scores greater than 30 have been linked to falls.[29]

INTERVENTIONS FOR MAXIMIZING FUNCTION AND MOBILITY IN OLDER ADULTS

The geriatric research literature is replete with evidence that indicates the benefits of regular physical activity and exercise in older adults, including stress reduction, diabetes control, reduced pain from osteoarthritis, and many others.[30] Interventions used by nurses caring for older adults to maximize their physical function and mobility center on first determining their baseline pattern, goals of the older adult, as well as available resources, motivation of the patient, and staff engagement. Although there is a growing body of research on the effects of physical activity with regard to improved health and function, improvement in geriatric syndromes such as falling, urinary incontinence and cognitive impairment, reduction in fear of falling, and improved quality of life, only a few are highlighted. Many of the interventions have been launched based on the seminal work of Resnick,[31] who demonstrated use of self-efficacy theory to foster improvement in function and physical activities in older adults.

Early Mobility and Walking Programs

For medically stable older adults, early mobility is essential to thwart functional decline in ambulation. Early mobility is an essential and basic aspect of care for all older adults. Recommendations for reducing functional decline include encouraging activity during hospitalization with structured exercise, progressive resistance strength training, and walking programs in coordination with rehabilitation.[32] Whenever possible, nurses should encourage older adults to get out of bed. Many different aids for the bedside are available to help assist the older adult to independently transition to a seated and standing position. Encouraging the older adult to walk short distances such as to the toilet with assistance is more proactive for encouraging mobility than encouraging the use of a bedpan or bedside commode. Nurse's aides can offer arm-in-arm or standby assistance to residents who are encouraged to walk on the unit. In some situations, use of a straight cane or walker may be required, but this can best be determined through an occupational or physical therapist evaluation.[33] In long-term care facilities, chairs are placed in the corridor to allow the older adult rest periods. Tracking the older adult's distance walked each shift is also important in order to realize the goals, which are set by the older adult and the nurse. Sharing this communication is also a fundamental role of nurses as they engage the older adult to continue to ambulate.

Quality improvement programs in acute care hospitals have also recognized the benefit of early mobility to prevent functional decline in their in-patient population of older adults. In one acute care hospital's intensive care unit, patients who received a mobility intervention has significantly fewer falls, geriatric syndromes, and catheter-associated urinary tract infections than those who did not receive the mobility intervention. The intervention groups also had lower hospital costs, fewer delirium days, and improved functional independence. Overall, the mobility group was out of bed 2.5 more days than patients in the routine care in an intensive care unit.[34]

Models of Care for Older Adults at High Risk for Functional Decline

Resnick's function-focused care[35] was created with the goals of optimizing function and physical activity among older adults who are hospitalized or residing in long-term care settings, such as assisted living, many of whom are experiencing reduced mobility and functional decline. Pre-discharge versus post-discharge results have shown greater improvement in older adults' function compared with control groups when used in the hospital for orthopedic patients, and when used in assisted living facilities, there is evidence of enduring changes and policies that support function-focused care.[36] In other related applications, person-centered mobility care practice in nursing homes has been used effectively to train staff, engage in weekly mobility care huddles, and reflective practice using motivational interviewing strategies over several weeks.[37] The seminal work of Naylor and colleagues[38] in their Transitional Care Model has noted improvements in health status and quality-of-life measures for chronically ill older adults as well as reduction in e-hospitalizations and costs when they receive care by a nurse-led interdisciplinary team approach.[39] Other national models shown effective in preventing functional decline include the Geriatric Resources for Assessment and Care of Elders (GRACE) model of Counsell and colleagues,[40] which uses an interdisciplinary intervention consisting of a nurse practitioner and social worker in coordination with the older adults primary care providers and geriatrics interdisciplinary team.

Wii Fit Exergames

The physical and psychosocial effects of the use of the Wii Fit Exergames, which were part of health education program, were studied and found that after a 4-week intervention, those elderly participants in the Wii Fit group experienced significant improvements in balance, mobility, and depression scores than controls. Wii Fit Exergames are commercially available and often used in long-term care communities to engage older residents in exercise.[41]

Yoga

Yoga consists of a series of practices or disciplines of the mind, body, and spirit that promotes flexibility, balance, strength, and endurance. Although its use originated centuries ago in ancient India, its use has been studied for its effects on symptoms and physical function among adults with chronic illnesses, such as osteoarthritis. Using yoga as an intervention, researchers found participants who engaged in sessions ranging from 45 to 90 minutes per session for 6 to 12 weeks experienced reduction in osteoarthritis pain, stiffness, and swelling.[42] Other evidence has found the use of yoga to improve pain and functional outcomes associated with a range of musculoskeletal conditions.[43]

Tai Chi: Moving for Better Balance

In randomized controlled trials of community-based programs for falls reduction, the risk of falling from use of tai chi intervention has been shown to be approximately 55% compared with control groups.[44] Tai chi is also reported to improve cognition in addition to physical function in older adults.[45] Tai chi has also been studied for its effects on functional decline and mobility. In a randomized controlled trial, tai chi was found beneficial to improve balance and cognitive performance in the elderly. Use of the FES showed improved scores in the group randomized to 6 months of tai chi training versus the control group receiving standard care.[46]

SUMMARY

Individualizing care to improve function and mobility is an essential component in the provision of quality health care to older adults. The overall health promotion effects of early intervention around a basic necessity, mobility, are clear. Untoward health outcomes from reduced mobility and functional decline are also well established. Professional nurses will need to advocate for older adults on their units in the hospital and in other settings, by critically analyzing policies and procedures, ensuring that mobility is properly assessed and mobility impairment is addressed by all members of the health care team. Use of models for care such as the Transitional Care Model, Function-Focused Care, and GRACE, as well as other established programs, have shown their clinical benefit to older adults with chronic illness who are at risk for functional decline. At center stage in these models are professional nurses and advanced practice nurses working within an interdisciplinary team approach. All nurses caring for older adults are stakeholders in the mission to improve the function, mobility, and overall quality of life for their patients by implementing evidence-based practice approaches and policies within their health care organizations.

Additional resources, tool kits, videos, and educational resources for nurses caring for older adults can be found on the Hartford Center for Geriatric Nursing, Try This Series, and ConsultGeriRN.

REFERENCES

1. National Center for Injury Control and Prevention (NCIPC). Available at: http://www.cdc.gov/HomeandRecreatonalSafety?falls/nursing.html. Accessed June 8, 2017.
2. Brown CJ, Flood KL. Mobility limitation in the older patient: a clinical review. JAMA 2013;310(11):1168–77.
3. Covinsky KE, Pierluissi E, Johnston B. Hospitalization-associated disability: "she was probably able to ambulate, but I'm not sure". JAMA 2011;306(16):1782–93.
4. Institute of Medicine. The future of nursing. Washington, DC: National Academies Press; 2011.
5. Gray-Miceli D. 2001. Changed life: a phenomenological study of the meaning of serious falls to older adults (UMI Microform No. 3005877).
6. Schwanen T, Ziegler F. Well-being, independence and mobility: an introduction. Ageing Soc 2011;31(5):719–33.
7. Inouye SK, Studenski S, Tinetti ME, et al. Geriatric syndromes: clinical, research and policy implications of a core geriatric concept. J Am Geriatr Soc 2007;55(5):780–91.
8. Costa AP, Hirdes JP, Heckman GA, et al. Geriatric syndromes predict post discharge outcomes among older emergency department patients: findings from the interRAI multinational emergency department study. Acad Emerg Med 2014;21(4):422–4333.
9. United States Department of Health and Human Services. Healthy People 2020. ODPHP Publication # B0132, November 2010.
10. Lunney JR, Lynn J, Hogan C. Profiles of older Medicare decedents. J Am Geriatr Soc 2002;50(6):1108–12.
11. Fried LP, Tangen CM, Walston J, et al. Frailty in older adults: evidence for a phenotype. J Gerontol A Biol Sci Med Sci 2001;56(3):M146–56.
12. Hart B, Birkas J, Lachmann M, et al. Promoting positive outcomes for elderly persons in the hospital: prevention and risk factor modification. AACN Clin Issues 2002;13(1):22–3.
13. Mick D, Ackerman M. New perspectives on advanced practice nursing case management for aging patients. Crit Care Nurs Clin North Am 2002;14(3):281–91.

14. Moore K, Boscardin WJ, Steinman MA, et al. Age and sex variation in prevalence of chronic medical conditions in older residents of U.S. nursing homes. J Am Geriatr Soc 2012;60:756–64.

15. Harris-Kojetin L, Sengupta M, Park-Lee E, et al. Long-term care providers and services users in the United States: data from the National Study of Long-Term Care Providers, 2013-2014. Vital Health Stat 3 2016;(38):x–xii, 1-105.

16. Frist WH. Overcoming disparities in U.S. health care. Health Aff 2005;24(2): 445–51.

17. Graf CL. Functional decline in hospitalized older adults: it's often a consequence of hospitalization, but doesn't have to be. Am J Nurs 2006;106(1):58–67.

18. Boltz M, Greenberg SA. Reducing functional decline in older adults during hospitalization: a best practice approach. Try This Issue No. 31 2012. Available at: https://consultgeri.org/try-this/general-assessment/issue-31. Accessed June 9, 2017.

19. Verbrugge LM, Jette AM. The disablement process. Soc Sci Med 1994;38(1): 1–14.

20. Melnyk BM, Fineout-Overholt E. Evidence-based practice in nursing and healthcare. A guide to best practice. 3rd edition. Philadelphia: Lippincott Williams & Wilkins; 2014.

21. Webber SC, Porter MM, Menee VH. Mobility in older adults: a comprehensive framework. Gerontologist 2010;50(4):443–50.

22. Gray-Miceli D, Ratcliffe SJ. Post-fall emotional responses, functional limitations and action plans to manage falls among independent residing older adults with recurrent falls. Gerontologist 2015;55(Suppl 2):644.

23. Kleinpell RM, Fletcher K, Jennings BM. Chapter 11. Reducing functional decline in hospitalized elderly. In: Hughes RG, editor. Patient safety and quality: an evidence-based handbook for nurses. Rockville (MD): Agency for Healthcare Research and Quality (US); 2008. Available at: https://www.ncbi.nlm.nih.gov/books/NBK2629/#ch11.ack1. Accessed June 9, 2017.

24. Centers for Medicare and Medicaid Services Releases: 2012 MCBS Access to Care Research Files: are Medicare beneficiaries getting the help they need with home-based care? Medicare current beneficiaries survey. Data Brief #002, 2014.

25. Pizzi LT, Toner R, Foley K, et al. Relationship between potential opioid-related adverse effects and hospital length of stay in patients receiving opioids after orthopedic surgery. Pharmacotherapy 2012;32(6):502–14.

26. Tinetti MD, Richman D, Powell L. Falls efficacy as a measure of fear of falling. J Gerontol 1990;45(6):329.

27. Centers for Disease Control and Prevention. Stopping elderly accidents, deaths & injuries toolkit for practitioners. Available at: https://www.cdc.gov/steadi/ Accessed February 1, 2017.

28. Berg KO, Wood-Dauphinee SL, Williams JI, et al. Measuring balance in the elderly: validation of an instrument. Can J Public Health 1992;83(Suppl 2):S7–11.

29. Podsiadlo D, Richardson S. The timed 'Up & Go': a test of basic functional mobility for frail elderly persons. J Am Geriatr Soc 1991;39(2):142–8.

30. Factora R. Aging and Preventive Health. 2013. Center for Continuing Education, the Cleveland Clinic. Available at: www.clevelandclincmeded.com/medicalpubs/diseasemanagement. Accessed June 8, 2017.

31. Resnick B. The theory of self-efficacy. In: Smith MJ, Liehr PR, editors. Middle range theory for nursing. 2nd edition. New York: Springer; 2003. p. 49–68.

32. American Academy of Nursing's Expert Panel on Acute and Critical Care. Reducing functional decline in older adults during hospitalization: a best practice approach. Medsurg Nurs 2014;23(4):264–5.

33. Quigley P, Goff L. Current and emergent innovations to keep patients safe. Technological innovations play a leading role in fall-prevention programs. Special report: best practices for falls reduction. A practice guide. Am Nurse Today 2011;14–7.

34. Fraser D, Spiva L, Forman W, et al. Original research: implementation of an early mobility program in an ICU. Am J Nurs 2015;115(12):49–58.

35. Resnick B, Wells C, Gali E, et al. Feasibility and efficacy of function-focused care for orthopedic trauma patients. J Trauma Nurs 2016;23(3):144–55.

36. Resnick B, Galik E, Vgne E, et al. Dissemination and implementation of function-focused care for assisted living. Health Educ Behav 2016;43(3):296–304.

37. Taylor J, Barker A, Hill H, et al. Improving person-centered mobility care in nursing homes: a feasibility study. Geriatr Nurs 2015;36:98–105.

38. Naylor MD, Bowles KH, McCauley KM, et al. High-value transitional care: translation of research into practice. J Eval Clin Pract 2013;19(5):727–33.

39. Naylor MD, Sochalski JA. Scaling up: bringing the transitional care model into the mainstream. Issue Brief (Commonw Fund) 2010;103:1–12.

40. Counsell SR, Callahan CM, Butter AM, et al. Geriatric resources for assessment and care of elders (GRACE): a new model of primary care for low-income seniors. J Am Geriatr Soc 2006;54(7):1136–41.

41. Chao YY, Scherer YK, Montgomery CA, et al. Physical and psychosocial effects of Wii Fit Exergames use in assisted living residents: a pilot study. Clin Nurs Res 2015;24(6):589–603.

42. Cheung C, Park J, Wyman JF. Effects of yoga on symptoms, physical function, and psychosocial outcomes in adults with osteoarthritis: a focused review. Am J Phys Med Rehabil 2016;95(2):139–51.

43. Ward L, Stebbings S, Cherkin D, et al. Yoga for functional ability, pain and psychosocial outcomes in musculoskeletal conditions: a systematic review and meta-analysis. Musculoskeletal Care 2013;11(4):203–17.

44. National Council on Aging: Falls free. Available at: ncoa.org/healthy-aging/falls-prevention/falls-free-initiative/. Accessed June 8, 2017.

45. Sun J, Kanagawa K, Sasaki J, et al. Tai chi improves cognitive and physical function in the elderly: a randomized controlled trial. J Phys Ther Sci 2015;27(5): 1467–71.

46. Nguyen MH, Kruse A. A controlled trial of Tai chi for balance, sleep quality and cognitive performance in elderly Vietnamese. Clin Interv Aging 2012;7:185–90.

Clinical and Community Strategies to Prevent Falls and Fall-Related Injuries Among Community-Dwelling Older Adults

CrossMark

Ruth E. Taylor-Piliae, PhD, RN[a],*, Rachel Peterson, MA, MPH[b],
Martha Jane Mohler, NP-C, MPH, PhD[b,c,d]

KEYWORDS

- Accidental fall • Accident prevention • Aged • Geriatric assessment • Injury
- Risk factors

KEY POINTS

- Falls are the leading cause of fatal and nonfatal injuries among older adults.
- Community-dwelling older adults should have an annual fall risk screening and/or assessment.
- Several evidence-based programs are available for community-dwelling older adults to raise awareness about falls, increase strength and balance, and address the fear of falling.

INTRODUCTION

As the aging population increases and lives longer, falls, fall-related injuries, and subsequent institutionalization are expected to increase. Various national studies from across the globe have demonstrated increasing fall-related incidence of injury (Canada), hospital admissions (Netherlands), and death due to falls (United States).[1–3] Preventing falls in community-dwelling older adults with, and without, a fall history is possible, but requires a multifaceted approach using education, clinical and community interventions, and health policies. The purpose of this article is to provide current evidence-based information on community-based fall screening, and comprehensive

Disclosure Statement: The authors have nothing to disclose.
[a] College of Nursing, University of Arizona, 1305 North Martin Avenue, PO Box 210203, Tucson, AZ 85721-0203, USA; [b] Arizona Center on Aging, College of Medicine, University of Arizona, 1807 East Elm Street, Tucson, AZ 85719, USA; [c] Division of Geriatrics, General Internal Medicine, and Palliative Medicine, College of Medicine, University of Arizona, 1501 N. Campbell Avenue, Tucson, AZ 85724, USA; [d] Mel and Enid Zuckerman College of Public Health, University of Arizona, 295 N. Martin Avenue, Tucson, AZ 85724, USA
* Corresponding author.
E-mail address: rtaylor@nursing.arizona.edu

Nurs Clin N Am 52 (2017) 489–497
http://dx.doi.org/10.1016/j.cnur.2017.04.004
0029-6465/17/© 2017 Elsevier Inc. All rights reserved.

clinical fall assessment, as well as community-based interventions addressing fall prevention. Falls may be similar in the community and nursing home; however, the relative rates and interventions differ in these settings. Thus, this article focuses on community-dwelling older adults. The authors address nonsyncopal falls (eg, falls that are not associated with loss of consciousness, stroke or seizure, or a violent blow).

Epidemiology

Falls are the leading cause of fatal and nonfatal injuries in older adults.[4] Each year about one-third of adults aged 65 years or older, and half of those aged 80 years and older, will fall.[5] Nearly half of all falls result in an injury,[6] of which 10% are serious,[7] and these injury rates increase with increasing age.[8,9] In 2015, direct medical costs for falls totaled $616.5 million for fatal and $30.3 billion for nonfatal falls in the United States.[5,10] Older adult falls can trigger a downward spiral in activities of daily living, independence, and overall health outcomes. Nearly 50% of older adult hospital admissions and most nursing home placements are a direct result of fall-related injuries, such as hip fractures, upper limb injuries, and traumatic brain injuries.[5,11,12] Although about 85% of older adult falls do not result in fracture or other serious injury, a prior fall is a significant risk factor for a subsequent fall, increasing the likelihood of injury from a future fall.[13,14] In addition, many older adults associate falls with a potential loss of independence; as a result, many community-dwelling older adults do not report noninjurious falls to their families or health care providers.

FALL RISK FACTORS IN COMMUNITY-DWELLING OLDER ADULTS

Falls in older adults are the result of a convergence of risk factors across biological and behavioral aspects of the person, and factors in their environments.[9] Risk factors for falling among older adults are generally classified as either intrinsic or extrinsic (**Table 1**). Falling is considered a "geriatric syndrome"—a "*multifactorial health condition that occurs when the accumulated effects of impairments in multiple systems renders an older person vulnerable to situational challenges.*"[15(p781)] In the United States, white older adults are significantly more likely than black older adults to suffer an injury because of a fall, which is likely due to lower rates of osteoporosis in African Americans.[16,17] Older women are likewise at a higher risk for injurious falls than are older

Table 1 Fall risk factors	
Intrinsic	**Extrinsic**
Advanced age	Lack of stair handrails
Previous falls	Poor stair design
Muscle weakness	Lack of bathroom grab bars
Gait and balance problems	Dim lighting or glare
Poor vision	Obstacles and tripping hazards
Postural hypotension	Slippery or uneven surfaces
Fear of falling	Improper use of assistive device
Chronic conditions (eg, arthritis, diabetes, stroke, Parkinson, incontinence, dementia)	Psychoactive medications

Data from CDC. STEADI: older adult fall prevention. 2016. Available at: https://www.cdc.gov/steadi/. Accessed December 5, 2016.

men, although aging men are more likely to have a fatal fall.[18,19] Low socioeconomic status, living alone, and social isolation have also been identified as contributing risk factors for falls among older women.[12,20] Physiologically, the risk of falling is increased with low body mass index, sarcopenia, and postural hypotension, as well as visual and hearing impairments.[21] Prior falls and fear of falling contribute to a cycle of diminished physical activity and muscle decline, thereby increasing the risk of falling.[22] In addition, undiagnosed acute illness, such as pneumonia or a urinary tract infection, as well as chronic illnesses, geriatric syndromes, and medication side effects all can underlie a fall event.[5]

Factors in the physical environment are implicated in about a third of all falls among older adults.[5] These factors can include poor lighting, loose carpeting, clutter, and stairs that do not have weight-bearing handrails for support. Unlike with youth and young adults, few falls in older adults are the result of engagement in sports or physical activity, but rather they more likely occur during activities of daily living in the home or community.[18,23] Specifically, falls occur most frequently when the older adult is transferring, or changing physical positions, such as from sitting to standing, climbing into a bathtub, or walking downstairs.[19] For many older adults, environmental factors are often downplayed because their environments have remained constant for a decade or longer. The increased risk in these environments is typically due to the physical decline of the older adult, leading to person-environment incongruence.[9,24]

SCREENING FOR FALL RISK

Older adults may think falls are a normal part of aging, or have concerns over institutionalization by overzealous family members, and may never report their falls to their health care providers or informal caregivers if they do occur. Thus, each time a health care provider does not screen for falls, there is a missed opportunity to prevent future falls. The American and British Geriatrics Societies' (AGS/BGS) joint Clinical Practice Guideline recommends that clinicians who care for older adults screen them for falls annually.[25] Initial screening can be easily performed at community health fairs, with primary care follow-up where indicated, or during primary care visits in the "Welcome to Medicare" or "Annual Medicare" visits. However, even during routine outpatient visits, a short and highly predictive question is to ask, "Have you had a fall in the previous 6 months?" If so, a follow-up appointment for a Comprehensive Clinical Fall Assessment should be made.

Comprehensive Clinical Fall Assessment

A multifactorial comprehensive clinical fall assessment coupled with tailored interventions based on the assessment findings can result in a dramatic public health impact, while improving older adult quality of life, as is recommended by the AGS/BGS joint Clinical Practice Guideline.[25] In response to this growing public health problem of falls among older adults, the Centers for Disease Control and Prevention's Injury Center "STEADI (stopping elderly accidents, deaths and injuries), Preventing Falls in Older Patients—A Provider Tool Kit" developed a broad, evidence-based resource designed with input from health care providers to help them incorporate fall risk assessment and individualized fall interventions into clinical practice with links to community-based fall prevention programs.[26,27] STEADI was developed through a comprehensive systematic review, which incorporated provider input of knowledge and practice gaps and contains an array of fall resources. The STEADI algorithm (see https://www.cdc.gov/steadi/pdf/algorithm_2015-04-a.pdf) begins with a 12-question "Stay Independent" patient self-assessment screening tool, with a score of 4 or more, or an affirmative response to any of 3 key questions (eg, fallen in the past year, feeling unsteady when standing or walking, or worried about falling) requiring additional assessments. These assessments include gait, strength, and balance testing, a vision examination, orthostatic blood pressure measurement, medication review, physical examination, cognitive screen, and a thorough falls history.[26,27] STEADI also provides care team information about falls, case studies, conversation starters, and video support and instructions for standardized fall risk, lower body strength and balance assessments (ie, Timed Up and Go (TUG) test, 30-second chair stand, and 4-stage balance test).[26,27] Patient and family educational handouts and fall prevention brochures are likewise available. All materials are open access and free of charge.[26]

EVIDENCE-BASED FALL PREVENTION INTERVENTIONS

For community-dwelling older adults, effective fall prevention has the potential to reduce serious fall-related injuries, emergency room visits, hospitalizations, institutionalization, and functional decline.[25,28] Evidence-based fall prevention initiatives should acknowledge the multifaceted risks for falling and take into account biological, behavioral, and environmental factors. In a recent systematic review[28] examining effective interventions for preventing falls among community-dwelling older adults, it was reported that group and home-based exercise programs, along with home safety interventions, reduced the rate of falls and risk of falling. In addition, multifactorial assessment and intervention programs reduced the rate of falls but not the risk of falling. Furthermore, Tai Chi was reported to reduce the risk of falling, whereas vitamin D supplementation did not appear to reduce falls.[28] Most guidelines reflect this and recommend that assessment for fall risk along with fall prevention interventions be multifactorial, based on the individual's fall risk.[25,29] At a minimum, it is recommended that assessment and intervention include vision screening, home environment, medication reduction, and exercise.[25] Additional evidence suggests the potential value in expanding upon these interventions to also include assessment and intervention for cardiovascular syncope and postural hypotension, osteoporosis, calcium and vitamin D levels, proper footwear, cognitive impairment, urinary incontinence, transferring skills, and providing hip protectors or other assistive devices when indicated.[11,25,29–32] More recent evidence points to the importance of dual-task balance training to reduce the risk of falling.[33] Although social factors, such as socioeconomic status and social isolation, are associated with increased fall risk, less evidence is available regarding the mechanisms for this relationship, or how to properly intervene in these areas to reduce fall risk. **Table 2** provides a list of sources for current evidence-based fall prevention recommendations.

SELECTED COMMUNITY-BASED EXERCISE PROGRAMS FOR FALL PREVENTION

Several community-based programs are commonly available for fall prevention. Different programs can raise awareness about falls, increase strength and balance, and address the fear of falling. **Table 3** provides information on what organization or organizations recommend these programs, and the evidential outcome of each. Some of the most common fall prevention programs are described below.

A Matter of Balance

A Matter of Balance (MOB) is a community-based educational program led by trained lay leaders,[34] which was developed by MaineHealth's Partnering for Healthy Aging (http://www.mainehealth.org/pfha). The overarching goal of the program is to reduce the fear of falling and increase activity goals for community-dwelling older adults aged

Table 2
Sources for identifying current evidence-based strategies for fall prevention among community-dwelling older adults

Source	Title	Publication Date	Type of Interventions Recommended
American Geriatrics Society/British Geriatrics Society, Panel on Prevention of Falls in Older Persons	Summary of the Updated American Geriatrics Society/British Geriatrics Society Clinical Practice Guideline for Prevention of Falls in Older Persons	2011	• Vision • Medications • Exercise • Home environment • Multifactorial
US Preventive Services Task Force	Prevention of Falls in Community-Dwelling Older Adults: US Preventive Services Task Force Recommendation Statement	2012 (update forthcoming in 2017)	• Exercise/physical therapy • Vitamin D supplementation
Centers for Disease Control and Prevention	A CDC Compendium of Effective Fall Interventions: What Works for Community-Dwelling Older Adults, 3rd Edition	2015	• Exercise • Home environment • Medications • Vision • Podiatric • Pacemaker • Multifactorial
National Center on Aging	Falls Prevention Programs	2016	• Exercise

60 years and older. MOB uses cognitive restructuring to manage concerns about falling.[34–36] During the MOB classes, a variety of strategies are used, such as restructuring misconceptions to promote a view of fall risk and fear of falling as controllable, setting realistic goals for increasing activity, changing the environment to reduce fall risk, and learning range of motion exercises to aid in fall prevention. Course content is provided through eight 2-hour sessions conducted once (8-week course) or twice per week (4-week course), during which participants learn problem-solving, skill

Table 3
Commonly available community-based fall prevention programs

Name of Program	Recommended	Program Goals	Evidence
A Matter of Balance	AOA, NCOA	Decease fear of falling and increase activity	Reduced fear of falling
The Otago Exercise Program	AOA, CDC, NCOA	Improve balance, strength, flexibility, and mobility	35% fall reduction
Stay Active and Independent for Life	AOA, NCOA	Improve balance and strength	Better balance, strength, and mobility
Tai Ji Quan: Moving for Better Balance	AOA, CDC, NCOA	Improve balance, strength, and gait	49% fall reduction

Abbreviations: AOA, Administration On Aging; CDC, Centers of Disease Control and Prevention[46]; NCOA, National Council on Aging (https://www.ncoa.org/healthy-aging/falls-prevention/falls-prevention-programs-for-older-adults/).

building, assertiveness training, and cognitive restructuring ("learning to shift from negative to positive thinking patterns, or thinking about something in a different way"), along with exercises to increase strength and balance. Participants of the MOB program report being more comfortable discussing their fear of falling and increasing their physical activity, and they would recommend the course to others.[34–36]

Otago Exercise Program

Developed in New Zealand, the Otago Exercise Program (OEP) increases balance and strength of community-dwelling older adults who cannot or will not attend a group-based exercise class. The OEP consists of 17 exercises performed in the home under the guidance of a trained physical therapist or nurse during 4 sessions, which are provided over 8 weeks with one "booster" session after 6 months. Participants are encouraged to do the exercises independently 3 times each week and to walk outside twice a week. Randomized controlled trials of the program have found on average a 35% reduction in falls among participants, including those with vision loss.[37,38] The highest benefits were found among those with the strictest adherence to the program, and those aged 80 and older who had experienced a fall in the prior year.[38,39] Implementation of the OEP across 8 states (ie, Colorado, Oregon, Pennsylvania, Connecticut, North Carolina, South Carolina, Nebraska, and New Hampshire) among 210 older adults (mean age = 80 years) resulted in significantly lower fall risk (TUG, $P<.001$), better lower body strength (30-second Chair Rise, $P<.001$), and better balance (Four-Stage Balance test, $P<.001$) following the 8-week program.[40]

Stay Active and Independent for Life

Stay Active and Independent for Life (SAIL) is a strength, balance, and fitness program for adults 65 years and older or those who have fallen, which was developed by the Washington State Department of Health.[41,42] The goals of SAIL are to reduce and prevent falls in older adults with fall prevention education and long-term structured exercise classes. Classes are conducted for 1 hour, 3 times per week by fitness, exercise science, or health care professionals who have completed the SAIL instructor training. The curriculum of activities in the SAIL program includes warm-up exercises, aerobics, balance and strength exercises, stretching, and education classes on falls prevention, exercise, medication safety, home safety, safe footwear, walkers, and canes. SAIL classes are able to accommodate people with a mild level of mobility difficulty (eg, cane user), because the exercises can be done standing or sitting. Every 12 weeks, a fitness check is completed on participants to assess fall risk (ie, TUG test), and strength (ie, biceps curl and chair stand).[41,42] Evaluation of the SAIL program among 91 older adults (mean age = 75 years) completing both baseline and follow-up testing found significantly better upper and lower body strength ($P<.01$).[42] Participants can attend SAIL indefinitely, because they are encouraged to remain active and independent for life.

Tai Ji Quan: Moving for Better Balance

Tai Ji Quan: Moving for Better Balance (TJQMBB), developed by Fuzhong Li, PhD, a Senior Scientist at the Oregon Research Institute,[43] is a research-based balance training regimen designed for older adults, people with balance disorders, or those who have fallen. TJQMBB is considered a functional therapy, based on Tai Chi principles derived from the Yang-style of Tai Chi integrating motor, sensory, and cognitive components to improve balance, strength, and gait, leading to fewer falls.[44,45] Participants in the TJQMBB program attend a 1-hour class twice per week for 24 weeks and learn a total of 8 core Tai Chi movements, along with a set of therapeutic movements. A minimum of 48 hours of TJQMBB is recommended to reduce fall risk in older adults. TJQMBB classes are taught by trained instructors and are able to accommodate individuals with a mild level of mobility difficulty (eg, cane user) because the movements can be done standing or sitting. Community-based implementation of the TJQMBB program in Oregon among 511 older adults (mean age = 75 years) across 32 senior centers led to a 49% reduction in the number of falls.[45]

SUMMARY

Most fall reduction programs are targeted to those known to have already experienced a fall. Given the low rate of reporting of noninjurious falls, a large portion of the at-risk population is never identified for fall prevention services. Nevertheless, the promotion of physical activity and home assessments can be easily implemented at a population level. The recommendations provided in this article equip nurses and other health care professionals with increased knowledge of current evidence-based information on fall screening, comprehensive clinical fall assessment, and community-based interventions addressing fall prevention in community-dwelling older adults. Although not every patient may warrant every assessment and intervention listed here, all older adults should receive targeted evidence-based fall screening risk assessment and intervention.

REFERENCES

1. Hartholt KA, van der Velde N, Looman CW, et al. Trends in fall-related hospital admissions in older persons in the Netherlands. Arch Intern Med 2010;170(10): 905–11.
2. CDC. Important facts about falls. 2016. Available at: http://www.cdc.gov/homeandrecreationalsafety/falls/adultfalls.html. Accessed December 5, 2016.
3. Public Health Agency of Canada. Seniors' falls in Canada: second report. Ottawa (Ontario): Public Health Agency of Canada; 2014.
4. Bergen G, Stevens MR, Burns ER. Falls and fall injuries among adults aged ≥ 65 years - United States, 2014. MMWR Morb Mortal Wkly Rep 2016;65(37):993–8.
5. Soriano TA, DeCherrie LV, Thomas DC. Falls in the community-dwelling older adult: a review for primary-care providers. Clin Interv Aging 2007;2(4):545–54.
6. King MB, Tinetti ME. Falls in community-dwelling older persons. J Am Geriatr Soc 1995;43(10):1146–54.
7. Tinetti ME, Doucette J, Claus E, et al. Risk factors for serious injury during falls by older persons in the community. J Am Geriatr Soc 1995;43(11):1214–21.
8. Schiller JS, Kramarow EA, Dey AN. Fall injury episodes among noninstitutionalized older adults: United States, 2001-2003. Adv Data 2007;392:1–16.
9. Stevens JA, Mahoney JE, Ehrenreich H. Circumstances and outcomes of falls among high risk community-dwelling older adults. Inj Epidemiol 2014;1(1):5.
10. Burns ER, Stevens JA, Lee R. The direct costs of fatal and non-fatal falls among older adults - United States. J Saf Res 2016;58:99–103.
11. Kannus P, Sievanen H, Palvanen M, et al. Prevention of falls and consequent injuries in elderly people. Lancet 2005;366(9500):1885–93.
12. WHO. WHO Global report on falls prevention in older age. Geneva (Switzerland): World Health Organization; 2007.
13. Sattin RW. Falls among older persons: a public health perspective. Annu Rev Public Health 1992;13:489–508.

14. Pohl P, Nordin E, Lundquist A, et al. Community-dwelling older people with an injurious fall are likely to sustain new injurious falls within 5 years–a prospective long-term follow-up study. BMC Geriatr 2014;14:120.

15. Inouye SK, Studenski S, Tinetti ME, et al. Geriatric syndromes: clinical, research, and policy implications of a core geriatric concept. J Am Geriatr Soc 2007;55(5): 780–91.

16. Kiely DK, Kim DH, Gross AL, et al. Fall risk is not black and white. J Health Dispar Res Pract 2015;8(3):72–84.

17. Curtis JR, McClure LA, Delzell E, et al. Population-based fracture risk assessment and osteoporosis treatment disparities by race and gender. J Gen Intern Med 2009;24(8):956–62.

18. Duckham RL, Procter-Gray E, Hannan MT, et al. Sex differences in circumstances and consequences of outdoor and indoor falls in older adults in the MOBILIZE Boston Cohort Study. BMC Geriatr 2013;13:133.

19. Tinetti ME, Doucette JT, Claus EB. The contribution of predisposing and situational risk factors to serious fall injuries. J Am Geriatr Soc 1995;43(11):1207–13.

20. Yoshida SA. Global report on falls prevention: epidemiology of falls. Geneva (Switzerland): World Health Organization; 2007.

21. Moreland JD, Richardson JA, Goldsmith CH, et al. Muscle weakness and falls in older adults: a systematic review and meta-analysis. J Am Geriatr Soc 2004; 52(7):1121–9.

22. Sattin RW, Lambert Huber DA, DeVito CA, et al. The incidence of fall injury events among the elderly in a defined population. Am J Epidemiol 1990;131(6):1028–37.

23. Tinetti ME, Williams CS. The effect of falls and fall injuries on functioning in community-dwelling older persons. J Gerontol A Biol Sci Med Sci 1998;53(2): M112–9.

24. Szanton SL, Roth J, Nkimbeng M, et al. Improving unsafe environments to support aging independence with limited resources. Nurs Clin North Am 2014; 49(2):133–45.

25. Panel on Prevention of Falls in Older Persons, American Geriatrics Society and British Geriatrics Society. Summary of the Updated American Geriatrics Society/British Geriatrics Society clinical practice guideline for prevention of falls in older persons. J Am Geriatr Soc 2011;59(1):148–57.

26. CDC. STEADI: older adult fall prevention. 2016. Available at: https://www.cdc. gov/steadi/. Accessed December 5, 2016.

27. Stevens JA, Phelan EA. Development of STEADI: a fall prevention resource for health care providers. Health Promot Pract 2013;14(5):706–14.

28. Gillespie LD, Robertson MC, Gillespie WJ, et al. Interventions for preventing falls in older people living in the community. Cochrane Database Syst Rev 2012;(9):CD007146.

29. NICE. Falls in older people: assessing risk and prevention. Manchester (United Kingdom): National Institute for Health and Care Excellence; 2013.

30. Tinetti ME, Baker DI, McAvay G, et al. A multifactorial intervention to reduce the risk of falling among elderly people living in the community. N Engl J Med 1994; 331(13):821–7.

31. Ungar A, Rafanelli M, Iacomelli I, et al. Fall prevention in the elderly. Clin Cases Miner Bone Metab 2013;10(2):91–5.

32. Moyer VA. Prevention of falls in community-dwelling older adults: U.S. Preventive Services Task Force recommendation statement. Ann Intern Med 2012;157(3): 197–204.

33. Agmon M, Belza B, Nguyen HQ, et al. A systematic review of interventions conducted in clinical or community settings to improve dual-task postural control in older adults. Clin Interv Aging 2014;9:477–92.
34. Healy TC, Peng C, Haynes MS, et al. The feasibility and effectiveness of translating A Matter of Balance into a volunteer lay leader model. J Appl Gerontol 2008;27(1):34–51.
35. Smith ML, Ory MG, Larsen R. Older women in a state-wide, evidence-based falls prevention program: who enrolls and what benefits are obtained? Womens Health Issues 2010;20(6):427–34.
36. Smith ML, Jiang L, Ory MG. Falls efficacy among older adults enrolled in an evidence-based program to reduce fall-related risk: sustainability of individual benefits over time. Fam Community Health 2012;35(3):256–63.
37. Campbell AJ, Robertson MC, Gardner MM, et al. Falls prevention over 2 years: a randomized controlled trial in women 80 years and older. Age Ageing 1999;28(6):513–8.
38. Campbell AJ, Robertson MC, La Grow SJ, et al. Randomised controlled trial of prevention of falls in people aged ≥75 with severe visual impairment: the VIP trial. BMJ 2005;331(7520):817.
39. Stevens JA, Sogolow ED. Preventing falls: what works - A CDC compendium of effective community-based interventions from around the world. Atlanta (GA): Centers for Disease Control and Prevention, National Center for Injury Prevention and Control; 2008.
40. Shubert TE, Smith ML, Jiang L, et al. Disseminating the Otago exercise program in the United States: perceived and actual physical performance improvements from participants. J Appl Gerontol 2016. [Epub ahead of print].
41. Shumway-Cook A, Silver IF, LeMier M, et al. Effectiveness of a community-based multifactorial intervention on falls and fall risk factors in community-living older adults: a randomized, controlled trial. J Gerontol A Biol Sci Med Sci 2007;62(12):1420–7.
42. York SC, Shumway-Cook A, Silver IF, et al. A translational research evaluation of the Stay Active and Independent for Life (SAIL) community-based fall prevention exercise and education program. Health Promot Pract 2011;12(6):832–9.
43. Li F, Harmer P, Glasgow R, et al. Translation of an effective tai chi intervention into a community-based falls-prevention program. Am J Public Health 2008;98(7):1195–8.
44. Li F. Transforming traditional Tai Ji Quan techniques into integrative movement therapy-Tai Ji Quan: moving for better balance. J Sport Health Sci 2014;3(1):9–15.
45. Li F, Harmer P, Fitzgerald K. Implementing an evidence-based fall prevention intervention in Community Senior Centers. Am J Public Health 2016;106(11):2026–31.
46. Stevens JA, Burns ER. CDC Compendium of effective fall interventions: what works for community-dwelling older adults. 3rd edition. Atlanta (GA): Division of Unintentional Injury Prevention, National Center for Injury Prevention and Control, Centers for Disease Control and Prevention; 2015.

Printed and bound by CPI Group (UK) Ltd, Croydon, CR0 4YY

03/10/2024

01040390-0012